THE CHINESE WAY TO HEALING

THE
CHINESE WAY TO HEALING

Many Paths to Wholeness

Misha Ruth Cohen, OMD, L.Ac.
with Kalia Doner

Illustrations by Robin Michals

A PERIGEE BOOK

Notice: The information in this book is true and complete to the best of our knowledge. It is not intended as a replacement for sound medical advice from a doctor. Only a doctor can include the variables of an individual's age, sex and past medical history needed for proper medical care. This book does not contain every possible factor relating to medical symptoms, illnesses or surgeries. Important decisions about treating an ill person must be made by individuals and their doctors. All recommendations herein are made without guarantees on the part of the author, the technical consultants or the publisher. The author and publisher disclaim all liability in connection with the use of this information.

A Perigee Book
Published by The Berkley Publishing Group
200 Madison Avenue
New York, NY 10016

Copyright © 1996 by Misha Ruth Cohen and Kalia Doner
Book design by Irving Perkins Associates
Cover design by Joe Lanni
Cover illustration: Arte cinese, Garofani; Free Library Philadelphia/Art Resource

First edition: September 1996

Published simultaneously in Canada.

The Putnam Berkley World Wide Web site address is http://www.berkley.com

Library of Congress Cataloging-in-Publication Data

Cohen, Misha Ruth.
    The Chinese way to healing : many paths to wholeness / Misha Ruth Cohen;
  with Kalia Doner.—1st ed.
        p.   cm.
    "A Perigee book."
    Includes bibliographical references.
    ISBN 0-399-52232-8
    1. Medicine, Chinese.   2. Alternative medicine.   3. Self-care,
  Health.   I. Doner, Kalia.   II. Title.
  R601.C69   1996
  610'.951—dc20   96-1390
                                                                     CIP

Printed in the United States of America

10   9   8   7   6   5   4   3

This book is dedicated to all my loving friends, clients, teachers, students, colleagues, and guides—as well as my adversaries. Each one of you has helped me to understand the intricate balance of Yin/Yang and to perceive wholeness as a continuous process, an unchanging state of perfection.

Particular mention goes to Stuart Kaplan, a client who came from L.A. to see me one time, but who, from that meeting, made it his business to turn my dream of a book into a reality. By introducing me to Charlotte Sheedy, he started the whole ball rolling.

I also want to express my affection and gratitude to Regula Noetzli, our agent, who saw the potential for this project and made it happen. And thanks to Eileen Cope, the editor whose initial interest shaped the project.

A deep bow of gratitude goes to the People's Republic of China, where great effort has gone into preserving the ancient art of Chinese medicine and bringing it into the twenty-first century. In 1987, a coalition of Chinese organizations invited me to come to China to speak on the use of Chinese medicine in AIDS treatment, and the Chinese have continued to try to deal with HIV/AIDS before it becomes a major public health crisis in China. This has been an inspiration.

Among my teachers, I'd like to mention Efrem Korngold; Andrew Tseng, my primary Chinese medicine teacher; Stuart Kutchins; Mutulu Shakur; all the teachers at Lincoln Detox Center; and those at the San Francisco College of Acupuncture and Oriental Medicine.

Deep appreciation goes to the doctors with whom I have worked who believe that the cooperation between Chinese and Western medicines holds great potential: Nancy Harris, M.D.; researchers Jeff Burack, M.D., Donald Abrams, M.D., and Robert Gish, M.D.; Silvio Schaller, Med. Arzt., Herr Professor Ruedi Luthy, M.D., and Rainer Weber, M.D., at Zürich University Medical School; plus the many enthusiastic lay people who have helped further the understanding between the two schools of medicine.

Thanks also to the staff of Chicken Soup Chinese Medicine; the board of directors, practitioners and staff of Quan Yin Healing Arts; and particularly to Cindy Icke, with whom I started Quan Yin. And to Shoshana Wechsler, Stanton Schaffer, Naomi Jay, Jeannette Egger, Iris Landsberg, Robert Goldstein, Isabelle Katz, Alfredo Baratti, Sadie Dawgh and Tosha Silver.

I am very grateful to those who contributed their expertise, time and support: Linda Robinson Hidas, Larry Wong, Abigail Surasky, Carla Wilson and Andrew Gaeddert.

This book is especially dedicated to all my family, especially my mother, Jackie, who fought cancer and illness for many years with great stoicism and finally died in peace; my grandfather Harold who, after his death, awakened me to the concept of death as simply another transition; my grandmother Ethel, who valiantly struggled with cancer before she died; my grandmother Lucille, who taught Yoga for many years and was rarely ill; my Aunt Jane, whose zest for life is a joy to behold; my father, Bart, who supported my early interest in science and lives life fully.

And I also dedicate this book to my dear friend Katharine Woodruff, a soul partner and psychic, who predicted this book long before its inception and has helped see it through all stages—from an idea, to its planning, conception, gestation, and birth.

And to Kalia Doner, without whom this book would still be only an idea. Our collaboration has truly been one of balance. And to Robin Michals, whose illustrations contribute so much to this book.

Finally, this book is dedicated to people living with HIV/AIDS, cancer and other life-threatening or serious illnesses who have accompanied me down this path. You have given me courage, encouragement, and knowledge. You have helped me open my mind and heart and live life to the fullest.

Contents

Preface

My Path

We are each traveling along our life path, being pulled inexorably toward our destiny, but so often that path is hidden from our conscious mind. We lose our way. Looking back, I see that my path to pursuing wholeness began when I was a child. I have always considered myself a scientist; even as a child, science and medicine fascinated me. When I was nine, a newspaper published a poem I'd written:

> Science is a wonderful thing,
> It can tell you how to talk and sing,
> It can tell you how a bell can ring.
> It tells you how birds can fly,
> It tells you how far is high.
> There are many more things I could tell you,
> Don't you think science is interesting too?

But it's a long way from the curious child to becoming a doctor of Chinese medicine. I took many detours and traveled many roads.

My grandmother, who my family thought was eccentric, was a vegetarian and a fruitarian, took daily walks for miles on Miami Beach, and practiced Yoga. When I stayed with her on the weekends, she would feed me soaked black mission figs and dried millet for breakfast. She started me on my journey, but I wandered off the path more than once.

When I went to college in 1969, the intensity of the times, my poor diet, and lack of sleep all contributed to a breakdown. I became chronically ill. The doctors I saw had no idea what was causing my malaise and the pain in my lower abdomen. Tests for mononucleosis were negative, yet I remained debilitated. Finally, three surgeons determined I had low-grade appendicitis and decided to remove my appendix. What they found were hugely swollen glands around the appendix area and announced that I did not have appendicitis after all; I had mononucleosis. Yet, they were baffled by the negative mono tests. I know now that I suffered from chronic fatigue immune dysfunction syndrome, a viral infection, but twenty-five years ago, it had not yet been identified by Western doctors.

It took me a year to regain some semblance of wellness after that gruesome experience and that struggle made me resolve to avoid having surgery again. I became a vegetarian and began learning about Western herbs and natural food therapy. My ideas about safeguarding the body's well-being were germinated by my grandmother's interest in diet and Yoga and grew as a result of my unfortunate encounter with Western doctors, but I wasn't focused in my quest. I still had many rough spots to travel along my path, none rougher than what happened on Route 80 in the winter of 1973.

Driving through a blinding snowstorm in Pennsylvania, on my way to settle in New York City, I was broadsided by a truck. I was unconscious for almost twenty-four hours. Five days later, I was out of the hospital and living in New York. I struggled to piece together a new life in a new town. My spirit was determined to succeed, but my body was suffering from the repercussions of the accident. I developed a tingling in my right leg. Luckily, I had a friend from the South Bronx who knew more about how to take care of such ailments than I—or my doctors— did. He was an acupuncturist. He felt my pulse, looked at my tongue, felt my back, asked me a lot of questions, and told me that if I weren't careful, I would have back pain very shortly.

As he predicted, I began to have searing, hot pain in my leg and back. I couldn't lift anything. I went to an orthopedist. He told me to lie down for three weeks until I was better. Three weeks later I was no better. Then I remembered that my grandmother had used a chiropractor as her primary care physician. I decided to give it a try.

My condition seemed to stabilize, but I still had a lot of pain. Weak and worn out, the chronic fatigue resurfaced. Often, I couldn't sit up for more than five minutes at a time.

Frustrated by my inability to help myself, I began to open up to alternative solutions. A friend kept telling me to try something called Shiatsu. Skeptically, I decided to go to a Jewish man with an Indian name who practiced Japanese massage. After the first treatment, much of the pain I had since the beginning of my back problem went away. I thought, "Hmmmm, there must be something to this." I reawakened to information and insights I had in college when I became a vegetarian.

I enrolled in a Shiatsu class where I learned about such things as Chinese and Japanese channel theory, pulse taking, moxibustion therapy, as well as how to perform a wonderful massage in the Japanese Shiatsu style. I also began to learn about the dietary theories of Yin and Yang.

My strength returned.

I started to practice Shiatsu, and after much agonizing, I took the risk of giving up a good job as an offset printer in downtown Manhattan. I soon had a thriving Shiatsu practice in Brooklyn.

My next leap in understanding of Oriental medicine came when Walter, the acupuncturist I'd consulted for my tingling leg, asked me if I would be interested in coming to an acupuncture school he was helping to set up primarily for African-American and Latino people in the South Bronx. It was affiliated with Lincoln Detox, well-known for its aggressive nonbelief in methadone and strong belief in self-empowerment for the people it served. Knowing nothing about acupuncture, I went.

When Mutulu Shakur, the head teacher, began to speak, I immediately knew I was in the right place. This was the beginning of my commitment to Chinese medicine. There was no turning back.

I studied and practiced Asian medicine—Shiatsu and acupuncture—until I moved from New York to California in 1979.

San Francisco didn't have any schools of Chinese medicine at that time, and the state of California would not recognize my New York training or experience, so, in 1980, when the San Francisco College of Acupuncture and Oriental Medicine opened its doors, I was the first student in the first class and the only one in that class who completed school and sat for the state boards. I became licensed in Florida in 1982 and in California in 1983.

It was between 1980 and 1982 that I saw my first patients with gay related immune dysfunction (GRID), often not even knowing what I was seeing. Then, in 1983, I went into private practice. Western doctors began to send me AIDS patients with only two to three weeks to live. There was nothing more they could do for them. I realized that although I felt compassion for these people, my heart was not as open as it could be. There was something within me that was afraid. This was very disturbing to me, and I needed to search within myself to cope with it.

The first thing I realized was that these people with AIDS made me remember the people I had known who had died terrible deaths from cancer as I was growing up.

I had a lifelong friend who was one month older than I. When we were nineteen, he developed bone cancer. No one told him that he was going to die (they believed it was better to keep such news from patients), but he knew. He confided in me: "I know that I am going to die but no one will tell me."

Then my beloved grandfather became ill with kidney cancer. He was in the same hospital as I was when the doctors operated on me for "appendicitis." I will never forget the day he called from a lower floor of the hospital and yelled into the phone that he wanted to see me before he died. The nurses would not let me off the floor, despite my ranting and raving. I tried to reach my doctor for permission, but he didn't call back in time. Finally, I was allowed to go, but only after my grandfather had lapsed into a coma.

I returned to college after my operation and his death and began to have dreams of my grandfather. This went on for three weeks. He would sit up in his coffin among beautiful flowers and fruit and talk to me. I don't know exactly what he talked with me about, but after that, I felt that dying was a transition, not an end.

These experiences deeply affected me. I also knew that the Western medical system was far from perfect and that the dying process in the United States was barbaric, especially within hospitals.

Realizing that these experiences were the source of my difficulties in dealing with the dire needs of my AIDS patients, I decided that I could not continue to treat people until I had done some internal work. I attended a five-and-a-half-day retreat on death and dying conducted by Stephen Levine and Jack Kornfield. They focused on silent meditation.

At the retreat, I became more and more aware of my own fear: not of dying itself, but of dying a terrible death. Slowly, with their guidance, I was able to come to grips with this fear, learning to be aware of myself and my feelings as I worked with others, especially those who are extremely ill. This lesson has allowed me to remain open to all people and their illnesses without having any sense of being burned out.

I cofounded Quan Yin Acupuncture and Herb Center in 1984 and in 1986, I received my doctorate in Oriental medicine (OMD) in gynecology from the San Francisco College of Acupuncture and Oriental Medicine. My goal was to create a community clinic for everyone, regardless of social status, ability to pay, or what disease they might have. I began to work more passionately and openly to develop programs for people with AIDS, who were shunned by most practitioners at the time. And it is people with HIV/AIDS, along with those with CFIDS, cancer, and chronic viral hepatitis, who have inspired me to make leaps that I might have never made on my own, who opened the doors of understanding and compassion and heightened my sense of the preciousness of the present.

Each one of our paths is unique. My path led me through illness, accidents, and life-transforming events to greater health and balance, becoming a healer and a teacher of healing practices.

Your path may take you anywhere. There may be many turns or roadblocks. Sometimes the path may disintegrate before your eyes. Yet, when you go inside yourself and pay close attention, you can visualize the internal path and that allows you to continue on the external one, just a little bit farther, one step at a time.

MISHA RUTH COHEN

THE CHINESE WAY TO HEALING

PART ONE

A Context for Healing

CHAPTER ONE

The New Medicine

Creating Your Own Path to Wholeness

Gwen wouldn't take no for an answer. She refused to believe: "No, we can't figure out what's causing your nausea and pain." "No, we can't do much for your depression besides give you drugs."

She initially came to the Chicken Soup Chinese Medicine clinic to enlist our help with her gynecological problems. For six months she worked with me, using acupuncture and herbs, to ease the monthly pain and nausea. "From the beginning, I could feel the improvement, but it still sort of snuck up on me, just how much of a difference it was making," says Gwen. After several months of weekly treatments, she no longer had to miss a day of work every month. She rarely had any discomfort, and pain was a thing of the past.

Gwen was pleased that she'd sought out a solution—and that it had worked. She'd been bouncing from doctor to doctor for years, and they never found a reason for her complaints. But Chinese medicine looked at her mind/body/spirit, not one isolated part of her body, and offered her treatments based on an understanding of her whole being.

However, despite her improved gynecological health, she was spiraling into depression. Her much-loved brother was diagnosed with HIV/AIDS, and she felt helpless and angry that she couldn't do more for him. She had trouble sleeping, she lacked energy, and she had lost interest in doing activities that she used to enjoy. "I couldn't think of how to do anything helpful. It all seemed useless," she says now, looking back on her sinking mood. "I guess I was always a bit troubled by depression, since my body had been out of balance for so long, but his illness pushed me over the edge."

Though she was scared, she didn't give up. She created her own path to wholeness by putting together a team of health care providers and making sure they worked together within the context of Chinese medicine's understanding of the unity of the mind/body/spirit.

"At first, I went to a psychiatrist for my depression. Then it occurred to me—I knew that acupuncture and herbs were effective; they cured my recurring gynecological troubles—maybe Chinese medicine combined with psychiatry could help my depression."

Gwen said that she wanted me to talk with the doctor so we could coordinate our treatments. She was in charge of her healing process; she guided us toward each other. The results were tremendous.

The psychiatrist and I compared diagnoses and treatment: I had determined Gwen suffered from Liver Qi Stagnation, which was causing the gynecological problems, and disturbances of the Shen, or spirit, which were producing depression. The doctor said Gwen was in a clinical depression and had decided she didn't want to take antidepressants. The doctor concurred with her and said it would help Gwen's growth if she could battle her psychological problems without drugs. That led the doctor to ask if I could provide treatment that would ease the physiological aspects of depression. I drew up a revised herb and acupuncture program and shifted the focus of Gwen's treatment from primarily the body to primarily the spirit.

Gwen then expanded her healing team to include several other practitioners. She used body therapy, both Feldenkrais and Rolfing, to quiet her anxiety and tension, and she began seeing a nutritionist to reshape her diet so it provided more energy.

In a matter of weeks, Gwen's whole demeanor changed. She began to believe that she might see some real improvement in her life. Her depression lifted. "Things are better now," she said at the time. "When I'm feeling bad, I don't think it's the end of the world. When I feel good, it doesn't worry me."

She's been directing her combined therapies for eight months now.

Her initial regime of acupuncture and herbs along with her weekly visits to the psychiatrist and the other therapies resolved the depression. "I feel terrific," she says. "It worked." For maintenance, she now receives acupuncture once every two weeks, takes herbs, and sees her psychiatrist once a month.

Gwen's determination to regain harmony in mind/body/spirit inspired her to create a comprehensive healing program. And it's to her, and to everyone who won't take no for an answer, that this book is dedicated.

The Chinese Way to Healing: Many Paths to Wholeness is your guidebook to pursuing health in mind/body/spirit. Using Chinese medicine as the great vessel that transports you toward wholeness, and bringing in many other healing arts as adjunct therapies, it demonstrates how you, like Gwen, can take control of your healing process and maintain or restore harmony in all aspects of your life.

This eclectic approach to healing, grounded in the philosophy and practice of Chinese medicine and embracing the wisdom and benefits of many other forms of healing, is what I call the *New Medicine*.

My belief in New Medicine evolved over the past two decades at my clinic, Chicken Soup Chinese Medicine, and at Quan Yin Healing Arts Center, of which I am cofounder and research and education director. In both centers of healing, our primary practice is based on Traditional Chinese Medicine (TCM), which is the consolidation of the ancient Chinese medical theories of acupuncture, herbal therapy, dietary therapy, and Qi Gong exercise/meditation. Our practice also harks back to the roots of Chinese medicine and places a great emphasis on treatment of disharmony in the mind, emotions, and spirit. Chinese medicine is the root of our healing approach because it provides a powerful way to view human beings in all facets of their physical and spiritual being.

THE POWER OF CHINESE MEDICINE

If you expand your concept of healing to include the Chinese way of thinking about the human condition, you may experience a subtle but powerful change in how you take care of yourself.

• Chinese medicine theory will give you a new way of describing illness. You don't catch a cold, you develop a disharmony.
• Chinese medicine will allow you to imagine a new way of overcoming illness. You don't kill a bug with a drug, you use acupuncture and herbs to dispel disharmony.
• Chinese medicine offers a new approach to treating physical problems and emotional upheaval. When you have a broken arm, you don't treat only the body. And when you have a broken heart, you don't treat only the spirit.
The mind/body/spirit is treated as a whole.

At the healing centers we don't recommend only Chinese medicine treatments. We encourage clients to use whatever other healing therapies are necessary to create balance, wholeness, and wellness. These therapies may come from Ayurvedic medicine, Tibetan medicine, standard Western medicine, homeopathy, chiropractic, Bach Flower therapy, body realignment therapies such as Alexander Technique, Pilates, and Feldenkrais, Therapeutic Touch, aromatherapy, the list goes on and on. These various modalities, joined with Chinese medicine and theory, are what create the New Medicine.

APPLYING THE NEW MEDICINE

You don't need to see a Chinese medicine practitioner or come to one of our clinics to reap the benefits of the New Medicine. There are many self-care techniques that can help you get started along your path to wholeness today. These techniques and therapies include Chinese dietary guidelines; various forms of meditation and exercise from Chinese Qi Gong to aerobics; Western nutritional supplementation, self- and partnered massages from Japan, China and the West; and soaks, saunas and compresses.

Self-care practices can make a dramatic and immediate difference in the quality of your life even before you have explored the Chinese medicine concepts on which the New Medicine is based. Self-care therapies are not second best. They're the most important part of any journey toward wholeness. You can't arrive there unless you bring yourself along.

THE BENEFITS OF NEW MEDICINE

The New Medicine offers the opportunity to maximize your pursuit of wholeness.

• You will have an opportunity to explore the basics of Chinese medicine philosophy and practices.
• You will learn about many self-care techniques that give you control over the harmony of your mind/body/spirit.
• You will become familiar with the comprehensive programs for general good health; management of digestive problems; handling stress, anxiety, and depression; breaking addictions; and managing women's gynecological health. They each set out a specific plan for using Chinese medicine, standard Western medicine, and various other Eastern and Western healing therapies to restore balance and harmony in the mind/body/spirit.

TAKING CHARGE OF YOUR PURSUIT OF WHOLENESS

Why did we develop this New Medicine that encompasses so many traditions and healing arts? Because many of my clients demand control over their healing process and access to the widest array of healthful therapies. It's their vision of healing that gave birth to the New Medicine and their determination that proved a person can move toward wholeness, even in the face of devastating illness.

About four years ago, a woman came to see me because she had been diagnosed by her Western doctor with endometriosis. She had emergency surgery, which made her symptoms worse, and she could not tolerate the proffered drug therapy because of her sensitivity to similar medication. She was extremely skeptical about Chinese medicine, but she was desperate to find some relief from the severe pain of her condition. I put her on a regimen of herbs, acupuncture, and nutritional supplements. Slowly, she began to become sensitive to how her body/mind/spirit were affected by the disease and could contribute to the cure. She began to meditate and practice visualization while we continued her healing regimen. After one year, she returned to her original Western doctor for an examination. He did another laparoscopy to check on the disease. There was no sign of endometriosis. She had combined Western and Chinese medicine and had both cured the physical disorder and propelled herself along a path to body/mind/spirit healing.

New Medicine can be a powerful healing tool when a cure, in a Western sense, is impossible. In fact, the people who I have seen become the most balanced and whole are not necessarily those who have become perfectly physically well. The most balanced are those who have gained maturity through growth and continual attention to the inner self. They may not have chosen to become ill, but they did exercise a choice about how they became well. Instead of allowing others to make decisions for them, they took control of their lives and their healing processes. Let me give you an example.

Nick, a client with AIDS, came to me in 1987. He had been diagnosed with lymphoma and was told by his medical doctor that he had two treatment choices: chemotherapy or no chemotherapy. When he asked what the results of treatment might be, he was told that with chemotherapy he could live six months but would feel horrible, and without chemotherapy he could live three to six months without feeling especially sick. Nick decided not to pursue any Western therapies for AIDS or cancer. He began a self-designed regimen of vitamin C and the use of crystals for healing.

When he arrived in my office six months after beginning his self-treatment, he challenged me to say what I could offer him. I said I could not necessarily extend his life, but I could offer him a healing process. My role would be to provide all the tools of Chinese medicine and, sometimes, the recommendation that he seek Western therapies. We started a program of acupuncture and herbal remedies, and he agreed to use Western treatments for the various syndromes and diseases associated with AIDS if it became necessary. I told him he would have to be part of the process. He agreed (not liking the Western part) and insisted that he must be in charge of his treatment.

At times, he listened to exactly what I told him; other times, he ignored me completely. At all times, he listened to his inner self, continuing to meditate and sit in front of his altar with all its crystals and objects that he found were healing for him.

Nick had one of the strongest spirits and the most irascible personality I had ever experienced. He lived for another five and a half years. This was a man who took full responsibility for his own healing and died a healed man.

These are but some of the paths to wholeness. As you search for your path, it is my prayer that *The Chinese Way to Healing: Many Paths to Wholeness* will help you along the way. Use the book as a resource. Take what you need and leave the rest. You may return to it again and again or sit with it and explore the deeper meanings in Chinese medicine. Your spirit will guide you. Healing will follow.

CHAPTER TWO

Understanding the Mind/Body/Spirit

Physiology and Anatomy in Chinese Medicine

Chinese medicine is a system of preserving health and curing disease that treats the mind/body/spirit as a whole. Its goal is to maintain or restore harmony and balance in all parts of the human being and also between the whole human being and the surrounding environment.

Each of Chinese medicine's healing arts—from dietary therapy and exercise/meditation to acupuncture and herbs—is designed to be integrated into daily life. Together, they offer the opportunity to live in harmony and to maintain wholeness. In fact, for all its power to heal the body, Chinese medicine's focus is on preventive care. In ancient China, doctors were paid only when their patients were healthy. When patients became ill, obviously the doctors hadn't done their job.

THE ROLE OF THE TAO

Chinese medicine's focus on maintaining wholeness and harmony of the mind/body/spirit emerges from the philosophy of the Tao, which is sometimes translated as "the infinite origin" or the "unnameable."

The guiding principles of the Tao are: Everything in the universe is part of the whole; everything has its opposite; everything is evolving into its opposite; the extremes of one condition are equal to its opposite; all antagonisms are complementary; there is no beginning and no end, yet whatever has a beginning has an end; everything changes, nothing is static or absolute.

This dynamic balance between opposing forces, known as Yin/Yang, is the ongoing process of creation and destruction. It is the natural order of the universe and of each person's inner being.

To Westerners, Yin/Yang is most easily understood as a symbol for equilibrium, but in Chinese philosophy and medicine, it is not symbolic. It is as concrete as flesh and blood. It exists as an entity, a force, a quality, a characteristic. It lives within the body, in the life force (Qi), in each Organ System.

Yin Organ Systems	Yang Organ Systems
Liver System	Gallbladder System
Heart System	Small Intestine System
Spleen System	Stomach System
Lung System	Large Intestine System
Kidney System	Urinary Bladder System
Pericardium System	Triple Burner (The Chinese medicine organ system that governs metabolism)

When the dynamic balance of Yin/Yang is disturbed, disharmony afflicts the mind/body/spirit; disease can take root.

Yin Disease	Yang Disease
This generally relates to Interior chronic conditions and is associated with:	This generally relates to Exterior disease located in the skin, muscles, or bone and it is associated with:
1. Pain in the body or trunk	1. Acute chills, fever, and body aches
2. Changes in tongue shape, size, and color	2. An aversion to cold or wind
3. No aversion to cold or wind	3. A thick coating on the tongue
4. A deep pulse	4. A floating pulse
5. Changes in urine or bowels	

Each symptom of Yin/Yang disharmony tells the trained practitioner about what's going on in the inner workings of a person's body. Once a disharmony is identified, the Chinese medicine practitioner addresses the entire web of interconnected responses in mind/body/spirit that are triggered by the presence of disharmony. Healing is achieved by rebalancing Yin and Yang and restoring harmony in the whole person.

APPLYING THE TAO TO PHYSIOLOGY AND ANATOMY

Chinese medicine not only conceives of wellness and disease differently from Western medicine, it also describes the internal workings of the body in ways you may not be used to. In place of individual organs or blood vessels and nerves, Chinese medicine identifies the body's Essential Substances, Organ Systems and channels.

These terms describe the internal working of the body in ways that are significantly distinct from Western ideas.

BASICS OF CHINESE MEDICINE ANATOMY AND PHYSIOLOGY

Essential Substances are those fluids, essences and energies that nurture the Organ Systems and keep the mind/body/spirit in balance. They are identified as: *Qi,* the life force; *Shen,* the spirit; *Jing,* the essence that nurtures growth and development; *Xue,* which is often translated as blood, but which contains more qualities than blood and transports Shen; and *Jin-Ye,* which is all the fluids that are not included in Xue.

Organ Systems, unlike the Western concept of organs, define the central organ plus its interaction with the Essential Substances and channels. For example, there is a Heart System, which is responsible not only for the circulation of what the West calls blood, but which also acts as the ruler of Xue and is in charge of storing Shen.

Channels, or meridians, are the conduits in the vast aqueduct system that transports the Essential Substances to the Organ Systems.

ESSENTIAL SUBSTANCES

The Essential Substances, which have an impact on and are impacted by both the Organ Systems and the channels, are called Qi, Shen, Jing, Xue and Jin-Ye.

Qi

Qi (*chee*) is the basic life force that pulses through everything in the universe. Organic and inorganic matter is composed of and defined by Qi. Within each person, it warms the body, retains the body's fluids and organs, fuels the transformation of food into other substances such as Xue, protects the body from disease and empowers movement—including physical movement, the movement of the circulatory system, thinking and growth.

We use the Chinese word for this substance because there is no precise English translation for the word or the concepts it contains. If you want to think of Qi as the energy that creates and animates material and spiritual being, the life force, or the breath of life, you will come close to understanding Qi. As you delve more deeply into Chinese medicine, you will begin to identify how Qi lives within you and fuels your very existence. You'll find Qi is most accurately defined by its function and its impact.

Where does Qi come from and where does it go? We are all born with Qi. We can preserve, create, or deplete it by the air we breathe, the food we eat and the way in which we live within our mind/body/spirit. There are many forms of Qi that all work together.

THE FORMS OF QI

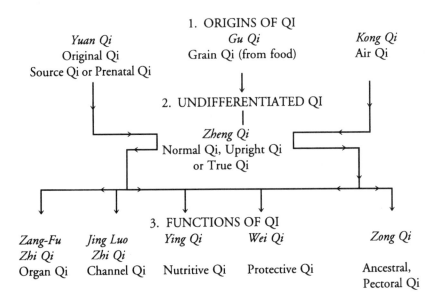

1. ORIGINS OF QI

Yuan Qi	*Gu Qi*	*Kong Qi*
Original Qi	Grain Qi (from food)	Air Qi
Source Qi or Prenatal Qi		

2. UNDIFFERENTIATED QI

Zheng Qi
Normal Qi, Upright Qi
or True Qi

3. FUNCTIONS OF QI

Zang-Fu Zhi Qi	*Jing Luo Zhi Qi*	*Ying Qi*	*Wei Qi*	*Zong Qi*
Organ Qi	Channel Qi	Nutritive Qi	Protective Qi	Ancestral, Pectoral Qi

Original Qi or Yuan Qi is transmitted by parents to their children at conception and stored in the Kidney System. It is partially responsible for the person's inherited constitution. We possess a fixed amount, which can be used up.

Grain Qi or Gu Qi is taken in with food, and it is released from the digestion of food in the stomach.

Air Qi or Kong Qi is extracted by the lungs from air we breathe.

Normal Qi or Zheng Qi is produced when Yuan Qi, Gu Qi and Kong Qi intermingle within the body. This is what is generally meant by the term Qi. It has five major functions.

1. Creates all body movement
2. Protects the body by resisting the entrance of External Pernicious Influences
3. Transforms food into Xue, Qi itself, plus tears, sweat and urine
4. Governs the retention of body substances and organs (contains everything and keeps it in its place)
5. Warms the body

Organ Qi or Zang-Fu Zhi Qi defines, influences and promotes each Organ System's proper functioning.

Channel Qi or Jing Luo Zhi Qi moves through the channels (meridians) bringing Qi to the Organ Systems and linking the Organ Systems and the Xue, helping them to function harmoniously. Acupuncture adjusts channel Qi.

Nutritive Qi or Ying Qi moves the blood through the vessels and transforms pure food elements into blood. It also moves with the Xue and helps it nourish body tissue.

Protective Qi or Wei Qi resists and combats External Pernicious Influences. It is the most Yang manifestation of Qi in the body. It moves within the chest and abdominal cavities and travels between the skin and the muscles. It regulates the sweat glands and pores, moistens and protects skin and hair and warms the organs. When Protective Qi is deficient, we are susceptible to the deleterious effects of environmental factors such as Cold or Wind, which are called Exterior Pernicious Influences.

Ancestral Qi, Pectoral Qi or Zong Qi gathers in the chest, where it forms the Sea of Qi. Ancestral Qi travels up to the throat and down to the abdomen and is responsible for breathing, speaking, regulating heartbeat and respiration. Meditation can strengthen Ancestral Qi and is particularly beneficial to maintaining or restoring harmony.

SHEN

Shen (*shen*) or spirit is as palpable to a Chinese medicine doctor as the heart or the left hand. Shen is consciousness, thoughts, emotions and senses that make us uniquely human. Its harmonious flow is essential to good health. Shen is transmitted into a fetus from both parents and must be continuously nourished after birth.

JING

Jing (*jing*) is often translated as essence, the fluid that nurtures growth and development. We are born with prenatal or congenital Jing, inherited from our parents, and, along with Original Qi, it defines our basic constitution. Acquired Jing is transformed from food by the Stomach and Spleen Systems and constantly replenishes the prenatal Jing, which is consumed as we age.

Prenatal Jing gives rise to Qi, but during our lifetime, as Jing changes, it is dependent on Qi. Qi is Yang; Jing is Yin. Qi and Jing are inextricably joined in the process of aliveness. While Qi is the energy associated with any movement, Jing is the substance associated with the slow movement of organic change. Jing is the inner essence of growth and decline.

Prenatal Jing is our genetic capability, but whether we reach our genetic capability depends on how much Qi we are able to nurture. Think of a child whose parents are six feet tall. If that child is malnourished, he or she will never reach the height conveyed by genetic potential. If there is an ample supply of food, then the child can grow fully. In the same way, if there is enough Qi, then the possibilities of Jing can become realized.

Prenatal Jing evolves through the stages of life. According to the ancient Chinese medicine text, the *Nei Jing,* in women, its changes accompany seven stages of life:

The Kidney energy of a woman becomes in abundance at the age of 7, her baby teeth begin to be replaced by permanent ones and her hair begins to grow longer. At the age of 14, a woman will begin to have menstruation, her conception meridian begins to flow, and the energy in her connective meridian begins to grow in abundance, and she begins to have menstruation which is the reason why she is capable of becoming pregnant. At the age of 21, the Kidney energy of a woman becomes equal to an average adult, and for that reason, her last tooth begins to grow with all other teeth completed. At the age of 28, tendons and bones have become hard, the hair grows to the longest and the body is in the top condition. At the age of 35, the bright Yang meridians begin to weaken with the result that her complexion starts to look withered and her hair begins to turn grey. At the age of 42, the three Yang meridians are weak above [in the face], the face is dark, and the hair begins to turn white. At the age of 49, the energy of the conception meridian becomes in deficiency, the energy of the connective meridian becomes weakened and scanty, the sex energy becomes exhausted, and menstruation stops with the result that her body becomes old and she cannot become pregnant any longer.[1]

The *Nei Jing* also states that men's development corresponds to eight stages of Jing:

As to man, his Kidney energy becomes in abundance, his hair begins to grow longer, and his teeth begin to change at the age of 8. At the age of 16, his Kidney energy has become even more abundant, his sex energy begins to arrive, he is full of semen that he can ejaculate. When he has sexual intercourse with woman, he can have children.

At the age of 24, the Kidney energy of a man becomes equal to an average adult with strong tendons and bones, his last tooth begins to grow with all other teeth completed. At the age of 32, all tendons, bones and muscles are already fully grown. At the age of 40, the Kidney energy begins to weaken, hair begins to fall off, and teeth begin to wither. At the age of 48, a weakening and exhaustion of Yang energy begins to take place in the upper region with the result that his complexion begins to look withered and his hair begins to turn grey. At the age of 56, the Liver energy begins to weaken, the tendons become inactive, the sex energy begins to run out, the semen becomes scanty. The kidneys become weakened with the result that all parts of the body begin to grow old. At the age of 64, hair and teeth are gone.[2]

XUE

The Chinese word Xue (*sch-whey*) is a much more precise description of this bodily substance than blood, which is the common English translation. Xue is not confined to the blood vessels, nor does it contain only plasma and red and white blood cells. The Shen or spirit, which courses through the blood vessels, is carried by Xue. Xue also moves along the channels in the body where Qi flows.

Xue is produced by food that is collected and mulched in the stomach, refined by the spleen into a purified essence (acquired Jing) and then transported upward to the lungs where Nutritive Qi begins to turn Jing into Xue. At the lungs, Jing combines with air and produces Xue. Xue is propelled through the body by Qi.

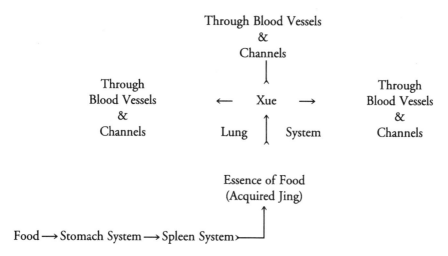

THE PRODUCTION OF XUE

Xue is intertwined with many bodily functions:

1. The Heart System rules Xue. Xue depends on the Heart System for its harmonious, smooth circulation.

2. The Liver System stores Xue.

3. The Spleen System governs Xue. The retentive properties of Spleen Qi keep Xue within its designated pathways.

4. Qi creates and moves Xue and holds it in place. The Chinese saying is, "Qi is the commander of Xue."

5. Xue in turn nourishes the Organ Systems that produce and regulate Qi. It is also said that "Xue is the mother of Qi."

MOISTURE/JIN-YE

Jin-Ye (*jin-yee*), the Chinese word for all fluids other than Xue, includes sweat, urine, mucus, saliva, and other secretions such as bile and gastric acid. Jin-Ye is produced by digestion of food. Organ Qi regulates it. Certain forms of what is called refined Jin-Ye help produce Xue. See the diagram on the following page for pure fluids.

These Five Essential Substances are the primordial soup from which life emerges and in which harmony and disharmony coexist. In Chinese medicine, reading the condition of these substances is an important part of diagnosis and treatment.

THE PRODUCTION CYCLE OF JIN-YE

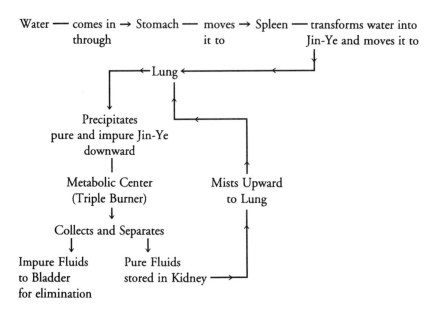

ORGAN SYSTEMS

Chinese medicine talks about Organ Systems—not the individual, anatomical organs that are identified by Western medicine. Although the Organ Systems are responsible for the organ functions that are familiar to Western medicine, they also embrace the organ's impact on the whole body. Each Organ System governs specific body tissues, emotional states and activities, and it is associated with and influenced by the Essential Substances and channels.

• Every Organ System is governed by Organ Qi and influences the balance of Qi. It is this energy that creates the Organ Systems' impact on the body/mind/spirit.

• The Essential Substances—Qi, Shen, Jing, Xue and Jin-Ye—infuse each Organ System with energy and shape its characteristics.

• Some Organ Systems are Yin and some are Yang. Together they are called the Zang-Fu Organs, and they form a harmonious balance that sustains life.

Zang (Yin)	Fu (Yang)
Heart	Small Intestine
Spleen	Stomach
Lungs	Large Intestine
Kidney	Urinary Bladder
Liver	Gall Bladder
Pericardium	Triple Burner

In general, Zang Organs are associated with pure substances: Qi, Xue, Jing, Shen, and Jin-Ye. Fu Organ Systems govern the digestion of food and the elimination of waste. But the division between Zang-Yin and Fu-Yang organs is not black and white. In the East there is no great compulsion to say, "This is X and it is always X. This is Y and it shall never be X." Each organ, whether Zang-Yin or Fu-Yang, has nourishing Yin and active Yang qualities within it. The dual unit of Yin/Yang exists within all life. For example, the Heart System stores Shen—that's a Yin function—but it also rules Xue, and that's a Yang function. The Liver System stores Xue, which is a Yin function, and it regulates and moves the Qi, which is a Yang function. This characteristic association with either Yin or Yang and with both Yin and Yang is true of each Organ System—and of Yin and Yang itself, which is the unity of opposites.[3]

THE ZANG ORGANS (YIN)

Kidney System

The Kidney System manages fluid metabolism, which the West associates with the kidneys and the adrenal glands. In addition, however, the Kidney System is responsible for storing surplus Qi and rules birth, maturation, reproduction, growth, and regeneration. The bones, inner ear, teeth, and lower back are also associated with the Kidney System, as is regulation of the growth of bone, marrow and the brain.

The Kidney System stores Jing and provides it to other Organ Systems and body tissue and is the root to eight important channels that connect the Organ Systems to one another.

The Kidney System opens up to the external world through the ear. Kidney harmony is revealed through acuity of hearing.

Spleen System

The Spleen System creates and controls Xue (as it is involved with the blood in Western medicine). It is also responsible for extracting Gu (Grain) Qi and fluids from food, transforming these substances into Ying (Nutritive) Qi and Xue and storing Qi that is acquired by the body after birth.

The Spleen System also maintains the proper movement of ingested fluids and food throughout the body. Gu (Grain) Qi and the pure fluids are transmitted upward to the Lung and Heart Systems by the Spleen System. Balanced fluid movement lubricates the tissues and joints. This prevents excess dryness and keeps fluids from pooling or stagnating and creating dampness. The Spleen likes dryness and is affected negatively by dampness. The Spleen System also is associated with muscle mass and tone and with keeping the internal organs in place.

When the Spleen System is balanced, the transformation and transportation of fluids is harmonious, Qi and Xue permeate the whole body, and the digestive tract functions well. The Spleen System's connection to the external world is through the mouth and the Spleen's vigor is mirrored in the color of the lips.

Liver System

The Liver System detoxifies the Xue and is responsible for the proper movement of Qi and Xue throughout the body. The Liver regulates the body by making sure Qi moves smoothly through the channels and Organ Systems; regulates the secretion of bile to aid digestion; balances emotions, protecting against frustration and sudden anger; and stores Xue. You can think of it as a holding tank where the Xue retreats when you are at rest. The Liver System also nourishes the eyes, tendons, and nails. The Liver System opens up to the world through the eyes and the health of the Liver is reflected in the sharpness of eyesight.

Lung System

The Lung System rules Qi by inhaling the Kong (Air) Qi from outside the body, which, along with Gu (Grain) and Yuan (Original) Qi, forms Zheng (Normal) Qi. As in Western medicine, the Lung System administers respiration, but it also regulates water passage to the Kidney System, which stores pure fluids. The Lung System also disperses water vapor throughout the body, especially to the skin, where it is associated with perspiration. In addition, the Lung System is in charge of Zong (Ancestral) Qi, which gathers in the chest, providing the Heart System with Qi. It also rules the exterior of the body through its relationship with Wei (Protective) Qi, providing resistance to External Pernicious Influences (see page 37). The nose is the gateway of the Lung System. The health of the Lung System is reflected in the skin.

UNDERSTANDING THE POWERS OF THE ORGAN SYSTEMS

Organ Removal

If an organ is removed (a woman may have a hysterectomy, for example), the body does not lose the entire Organ System or its contribution to the harmony of the mind/body/spirit: The energetics of the Organ System and its associated channel remain. Although the removal of an organ creates an imbalance, it can be addressed with acupuncture, herbs, dietary adjustments and exercise/meditation.

Intangible Organ Systems

In Chinese medicine, there is an Organ System—The Triple Burner—that you couldn't find if you were to cut open the body and search for it. This is possible because Organ Systems, like much in Chinese medicine, are defined by function, not location. The term *Organ System* in Chinese medicine describes a nexus of functions that are concrete and have identifiable traits. That's all the information that's needed to be able to chart the development of disharmony in an Organ System and to remedy it.

Heart System

The Heart System is associated with the heart, the movement of the Xue through the vessels, and the storing of Shen. It is the ruler of the Xue and the blood vessels. When the heart's Xue and Qi are in harmony, the Shen is at peace, and a person has an easy time dealing with what the world dishes out. The emotional states of joy or lack of joy, as well as charisma, are associated with the Heart System.

The Heart opens into the tongue and abundant Heart Xue is revealed by facial skin that is well-moisturized and supple.

Pericardium

The Pericardium is the covering or protector of the Heart muscle and provides the outermost defense of the Heart against external causes of disharmony. Although it has no physiological function separate from the Heart, it has its own acupuncture channel. It is considered a distinct Organ System because it disperses Excess Qi from the Heart and directs it to a point in the center of the palm where it can exit the body naturally.

THE FU ORGANS (YANG)

The Fu organs' main purpose is to receive food, absorb usable nutrition and excrete waste. Fu organs are considered less internal than the Zang organs because they are associated with impure substances: food, urine, and feces. Although this sometimes diminishes their importance, the Fu organs and channels play a major role in acupuncture.

Gallbladder System

Working with the Liver System, the Gallbladder System stores and secretes bile into the Large and Small Intestine Systems to help digestion. Any disharmony of the Liver System impacts the Gallbladder System and vice versa.

Stomach System

The stomach receives and decomposes food so the Spleen System can transform the fluids and food essence into Qi and Xue. The Stomach System is also responsible for moving Qi downward and sending waste to the Intestines. The Spleen moves Qi upward, and harmony between the Stomach and Spleen is vital.

Small Intestine System

Working with the Stomach System, the Small Intestine helps produce Qi and Xue. The Small Intestine separates and refines the pure from the impure in fluids, food, and in the mind.

Large Intestine System

Moving the impure waste down through the body, the Large Intestine extracts water and produces feces.

Urinary Bladder System

Urine, produced by the Kidney and Lung Systems and from intestinal waste water, is excreted by the Bladder.

Triple Burner System

This Organ System, which is divided into three parts—the Upper Burner, Middle Burner, and Lower Burner—does not exist in Western medicine. In Chinese texts it is called *Sanjiao* and is said to have "name without shape." The best way to understand the Triple Burner is to examine its function, which is to mediate the body's water metabolism. Don't worry about where it lives, but what it does.

The Upper Burner is identified in the *Ling Shu* as an all-pervasive, light fog that distributes the Qi of water and food throughout the body. This part of the Triple Burner is associated with the head and chest and the Heart and Lung Organ Systems.

The Middle Burner, identified as a froth of bubbles, is associated with the Spleen, Stomach and, according to some practitioners, the Liver. It's involved with digestion, absorption of Essential Substances, evaporating fluids and imbuing Xue with Nutritive Qi. The froth of bubbles refers to the state of decomposing, digested foods.

The Lower Burner, which is called a drainage ditch, designates an area below the navel and includes the Kidney, Large and Small Intestines, Bladder and Liver (due to the location of the acupuncture channel). It governs the elimination of impurities. The Lower Burner helps regulate the Large Intestine and helps the Kidney System to process waste.[4]

EXTRAORDINARY OR ANCESTRAL FU ORGANS

The Brain, Marrow, Bones, Blood Vessels and the Uterus, plus the Gallbladder System, are called the Extraordinary Organs. The ancient Chinese medical text *Nei Jing* states that they resemble the Fu (Yang) organs in form and the Zang

(Yin) organs in function. The marrow, which includes the spinal chord, Bone, and Brain are wedded to the Kidney System and their existence depends on Jing, which gives rise to Brain and Marrow. The Marrow nourishes the Bones.

The Brain

This is the Sea of Marrow and is nourished by the marrow. The five senses plus memory and thinking are associated with other Organ Systems, but they are influenced by the Brain. Consciousness is also associated with the Brain. Although the Heart stores the Shen, the Brain is also associated with it.

The Uterus

The uterus is called Bao Gong (palace of the child), and it usually functions as a storage organ. However, in relation to menstruation and labor, its function is to discharge. While it is the anatomical source of menstruation and the location of gestation, its functioning is governed by other Organ Systems.

Both the conception and penetrating channel rise from the uterus. Menstruation depends on these channels' harmonious functioning, on the strength of the Kidney Jing and on the Xue functions of the Spleen and Liver Systems. The uterus's reproductive function is dominated by Kidney Qi because reproduction is related to the Kidney. When the function of the Heart and Kidney Systems is balanced, menstruation is normal. When the Heart and Kidney functions are strong, conception is easy. Men are said to possess the energetic area of the uterus. It contributes to their harmony and affects the flow of Essential Substances through the conception and penetrating channels.

The Blood Vessels

The blood vessels transport most of the Xue through the body. Although the distinction between Xue circulating in the blood vessels and in the channels is not delineated, it's generally accepted that blood vessels carry more Xue than Qi and channels carry more Qi than Xue.

Understanding how the vessels function cannot be separated from understanding the relationship between the Xue and the Zang Organ Systems. Heart rules the Xue, keeping the heartbeat regular and balanced; the Liver System stores and regulates the Xue, keeping an even flow of Xue throughout the body; and the Spleen governs the Xue, keeping it within the vessels and channels. Disharmony of the blood vessels may be corrected by treating one of these Organ Systems.

The Gallbladder

The gallbladder is considered both a Fu Organ and an Extraordinary Organ because it contributes to the breakdown of impure food—a Yang function—but unlike any other Yang organ, it contains a pure fluid, bile.

THE CHANNELS

The channels, sometimes called meridians or vessels, are a great aqueduct system that transports the Essential Substances—Qi, Jing, Xue, Jin-Ye and Shen—to each Organ System and every part of the body. By tuning in to the way Qi moves through the body's channels, Chinese medicine practitioners can "read" the harmony or disharmony of the body's Essential Substances and Organ Systems. They can also manipulate the flow of Qi and other Essential Substances through the channels in order to keep the flow irrigating the body evenly.

Acupuncture controls the flow of the Essential Substances by needling acupoints that are positioned along the network of channels like a series of gates. At these points, the flow of Essential Substances, particularly Qi, comes close to the surface of the skin and the needling stimulates or retards their passage through the channels.

The functions of the channels, according to Traditional Chinese Medicine, are to:

1. Transport Xue and Qi and regulate Yin and Yang
2. Resist pathogens and reflect symptoms and signs of disease and disharmony
3. Transmit curative sensations that occur during acupuncture, such as the spreading of warmth and relaxation through the body, the sense of Qi moving, or a feeling of concentrated heaviness
4. Regulate Excess and Deficiency conditions

The major channels are divided into twelve primary channels, eight extraordinary channels and fifteen collaterals. There are also the less-often-discussed twelve divergent channels, the twelve muscle regions and the twelve cutaneous regions.

THE TWELVE PRIMARY CHANNELS

Each primary channel is linked to an Organ System, transports Qi and other Essential Substances and helps maintain harmony in mind/body/spirit. The *Ling Shu*, part of the *Nei Jing*, explains, "Internally, the twelve regular meridians connect with the Zang-Fu organs and externally with the joints, limbs and other superficial tissues of the body."

The twelve primary channels are: Lung, Large Intestine, Stomach, Spleen, Heart, Small Intestine, Bladder, Kidney, Pericardium, Triple Burner, Gallbladder and Liver.

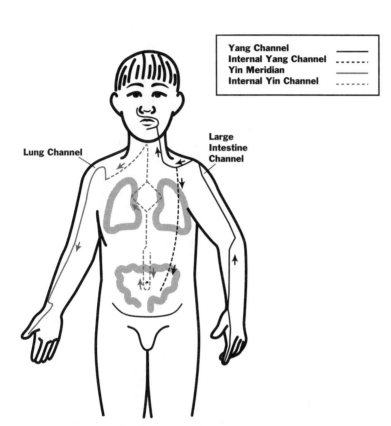

Lung Channel

Large Intestine Channel

Yang Channel   ———
Internal Yang Channel   -------
Yin Meridian   ———
Internal Yin Channel   -------

The Lung Channel of Hand-Taiyin
The Large Intestine Channel of Hand-Yangming

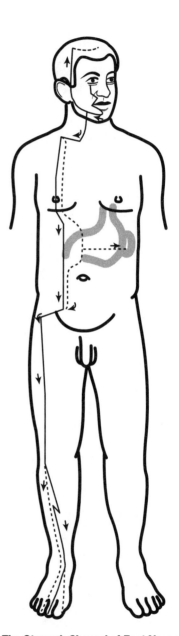

The Stomach Channel of Foot-Yangming

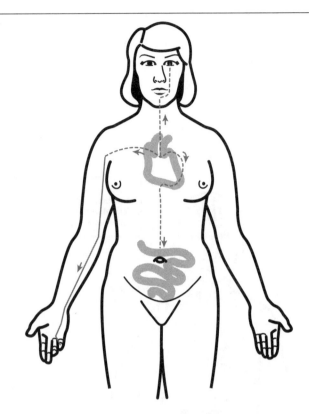

The Heart Channel of Hand-Shaoyin

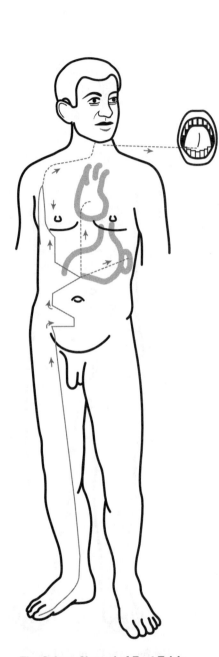

The Spleen Channel of Foot-Taiyin

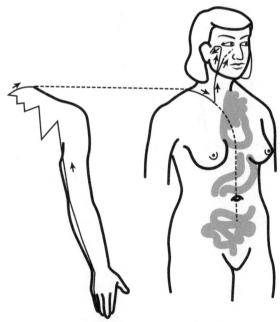

The Small Intestine Channel of Hand-Taiyang

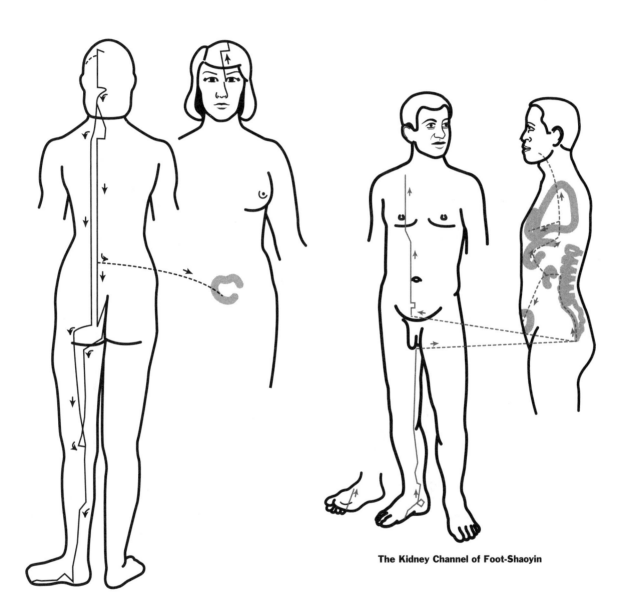

The Kidney Channel of Foot-Shaoyin

The Bladder Channel of Foot-Taiyang

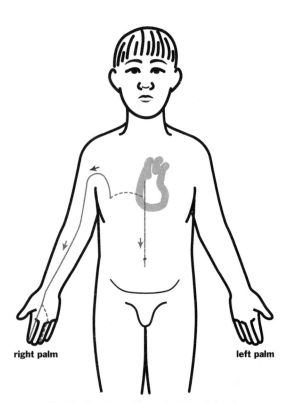

right palm   left palm

The Pericardium Channel of Hand-Jueyin

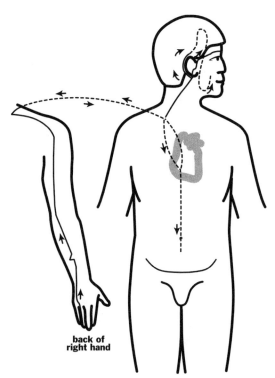

back of
right hand

The Triple Burner (Sanjiao) Channel of Hand-Shaoyang

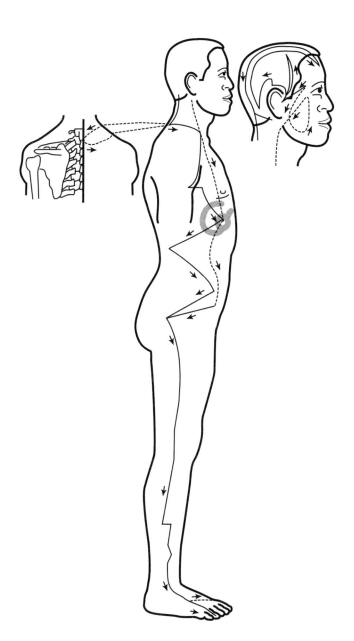

The Gallbladder Channel of Foot-Shaoyang

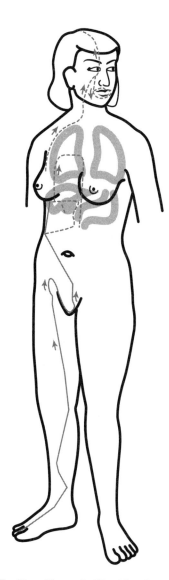

The Liver Channel of Foot-Jueyin

Each channel is defined by whether it starts or ends at the hand or foot; whether the channel is Yin (runs along the center of the body) or Yang (runs along the sides of the body); and whether it is related to a Zang Organ System (the Lung, Kidney, Spleen, Heart, Liver, Pericardium) or a Fu Organ System (Small Intestine, Large Intestine, Stomach, Gallbladder, Triple Burner).

THE CYCLICAL FLOW OF QI IN THE TWELVE REGULAR CHANNELS

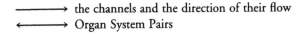

> ⟶ the channels and the direction of their flow
> ⟷ Organ System Pairs

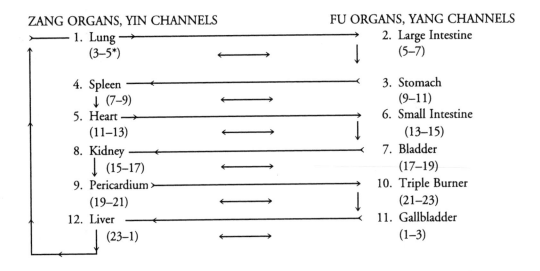

ZANG ORGANS, YIN CHANNELS   FU ORGANS, YANG CHANNELS

1. Lung ⟶   2. Large Intestine
   (3–5*)   (5–7)

4. Spleen ⟵   3. Stomach
   ↓ (7–9)   (9–11)
5. Heart ⟶   6. Small Intestine
   (11–13)   (13–15)
8. Kidney ⟵   7. Bladder
   ↓ (15–17)   (17–19)
9. Pericardium ⟶   10. Triple Burner
   (19–21)   (21–23)
12. Liver ⟵   11. Gallbladder
    ↓ (23–1)   (1–3)

Each Yin channel and Zang Organ is paired with a Yang channel and Fu Organ—the Lung and Large Intestine; the Spleen and Stomach; the Kidney and Bladder; the Pericardium and Triple Burner; and the Liver and the Gallbladder. This association means that if one of the paired organs becomes unbalanced, the other may be thrown into disharmony as well.

*The time of day when each channel is most open and active is noted under each organ (time given for twenty-four-hour clock).

EIGHT EXTRAORDINARY CHANNELS

In addition to the twelve primary channels, there are eight extraordinary channels. According to another ancient medical text, the *Nan Jing*, "The twelve organ-related Qi Channels constitute rivers and the eight extraordinary vessels (channels) constitute reservoirs." Unlike the primary channels, the eight extraordinary channels aren't associated with any of the twelve Organ Systems, but they are extremely important because they augment the communication between the twelve channels, act as a storage system for Qi and exert a strong effect on personality. These reservoirs collect Excess Qi, releasing it into the various primary channels if they become Qi Deficient because of mental or physical stress or trauma. They also have their own special functions. Some French acupuncturists call them "miraculous meridians" because they are used for therapeutic effects when other techniques prove ineffective.

Four of the extraordinary channels are located in the trunk of the body. These are solitary, unpaired channels with special functions. They are:

The Chong Mai

The Chong Mai (*chong-my*) or penetrating channel is also known as the Sea of Qi and Xue. It regulates the Qi and Xue of the twelve channels and distributes Jing throughout the body. In the lower body, the Chong Mai is one channel, but in the upper body, as it meets the Kidney channel, it splits into two forks that rise up each side of the chest. It brings the Kidney Qi upward to the abdomen and chest. The Chong Mai is the root of the other extraordinary channels.

The Ren Mai

The Ren Mai (*ren-my*) or Conception channel regulates the six Yin channels and Yin throughout the body. It's in charge of the Jin-Ye and Jing and regulates the supply of body fluids to the fetus. Along with the Chong Mai, this channel originates in the uterus, supporting and supplying the uterus and regulating the seven- and eight-year life cycles in women and men. (In men, the energetic area of the uterus exists even without the presence of the physical organ.)

The Du Mai

The Du Mai (*doo-my*) or governing channel also rises from the uterus and links the spinal cord and the brain and all the Yang channels. (The uterine area of the body exists in both men and women.) The Du Mai is the master of all the Yang energy. Along with the Ren Mai, it regulates the balance of Yin/Yang, which in turn regulates the balance of Qi and Xue.

The Dai Mai

The Dai Mai (*die-my*) or belt channel encircles the middle of the body like a belt. It links together all other channels and controls the Chong, Ren and Du Mai and strengthens their links to the uterus.

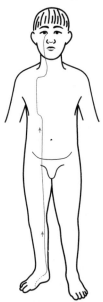

The Yinqiao Channel

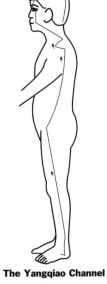

The Yangqiao Channel

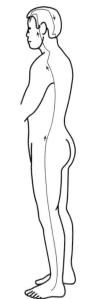

The Yangwei Channel

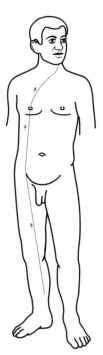

The Yinwei Channel

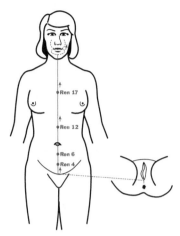

The Ren Channel

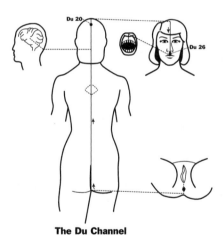

The Du Channel

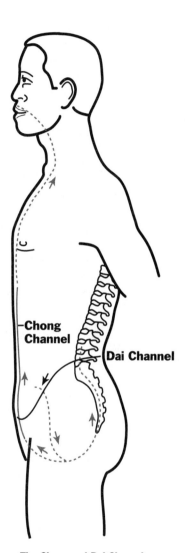

The Chong and Dai Channels

The last four extraordinary channels are located in the trunk and legs and are paired. They are:

The Yangqiao Mai

The Yangqiao Mai (*yang-chow-my*) or Yang heel channel connects with the governing vessel. The Qi supplying this channel is generated through leg exercises and rises upward to nourish the Yang channels.

The Yinqiao Mai

The Yinqiao Mai (*yin-chow-my*) or Yin heel channel connects with the Kidney channel. Qi enters the channel through the transformation of Kidney Jing into Qi.

The Yangwei Mai

The Yangwei Mai (*yang-way-my*) or Yang linking channel regulates Qi in the Yang channels, including the Du Mai. Yangwei connects and networks the Exterior Yang of the whole body.

The Yinwei Mai

The Yinwei Mai (*yin-way-mai*) or Yin linking channel connects with the Kidney, Liver and Spleen Yin channels, the Ren Mai and the Interior Yin of the whole body.

THE FIFTEEN COLLATERALS

These are branches of the primary channels. They run from side to side along the exterior of the body and have the same acupuncture points as the primary channels. They also take their names from the twelve primary channels plus the Du, the Ren and great collateral of the Spleen.

The collaterals are responsible for controlling, joining, storing and regulating the Qi and Xue of each primary channel.

FIVE PHASES: ANOTHER VIEW OF HOW THE MIND/BODY/SPIRIT WORKS

You may have heard of the Five Phases, or as they are sometimes called, the Five Elements. This is the philosophical basis for the systems used by the Worsley School acupuncturists and many Japanese and Korean practitioners to describe both the physiology of the mind/body/spirit and to guide diagnosis and treatment. Strictly speaking, Traditional Chinese Medicine (TCM) does not use the Five Phases for treatment, but many TCM practitioners also incorporate the phases into their diagnosis and treatment since many aspects of the Five Phases provide powerful diagnostic tools. I often use Five Phases–based treatment plans for problems that are primarily emotional or that I intuitively sense would benefit from the approach.

The Five Phases—wood, fire, metal, water, and earth—describe the dynamic system of matter's transformation through growth, decline, decay, rebirth, and balance. This continual cycle of growth and dormancy exists in both the external world and the world within human beings.

A person may be characterized as being predominantly wood or earth or fire or water or metal, or a combination of phases. A disharmony may manifest the influence of one or more phases as well.

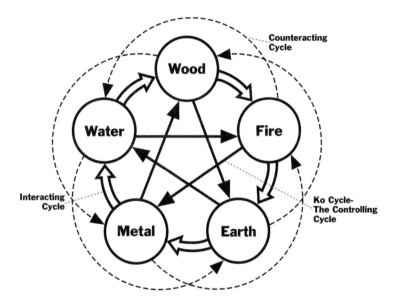

Around the outside of the illustration is the Shen cycle or cycle of creation: Wood burns fire, which, when turned to ashes, forms the earth, from which metal is derived, which in turn if heated becomes liquid, like water. Water then creates wood and the creation cycle is whole.

The destruction or Ko cycle connects the phases (see the arrows in the center of the diagram). This is the cycle that controls and balances the phases. Wood controls earth; earth controls water; water controls fire; fire controls metal; and metal controls wood.

The tension between creation and destruction and the interrelationship of the five phases maintains the natural flow and harmony. Disharmony in one phase impacts the associated phases.

Each phase is associated with and describes a stage of transition, a direction, color climate, human sound, emotion, taste, Yin Organ, Yang Organ, sense organ, tissue, smell and a grain. These associations aid diagnosis, providing detailed clues about the nature of disharmonies.

Emotions are of particular importance in the Five Phases system, and practitioners spend a great deal of time in their initial interview with a client, asking about the Seven Emotions: joy, anger, grief, sadness, fear, fright, and meditation. Every disharmony or illness in a Phase is associated with an emotion. That emotion is a strong indication of where in the body to look for illness and which channels to treat with acupuncture. The Five Phases practitioner will also evaluate facial colors, smell, touch, and pulses, although these are sometimes different in character from TCM.[5] Each phase is associated with acupuncture channels, and disharmony in a phase or phases indicates which channel(s) to treat to help restore harmony.

To help you understand how the Five Phases system translates into practical medical care, you may want to familiarize yourself with the basic principles.

Wood is associated with functions in the growing stage of life. Like a strong, rooted tree that grows upward and outward, a wood person is firmly anchored with a clear, strong Qi. If the Qi is not clear, you feel off-balance, uprooted. Your limbs are not nourished by sufficient Qi. You may have spinal problems.

The Liver System, associated with wood, governs the flow of Qi. People who are Liver dominant are critical thinkers and problem solvers, well-focused, and take charge of business. The psychic sense of Liver is that it carries things into the future. When Liver is overdominant a person may become compulsive, rigid, irritable, and judgmental. The Gallbladder is also associated with wood. It is also related to the decision-making ability.

The emotion of anger is wood and can be excess or deficient. The climate connected with the Liver is wind, and that has an impact on health because, as the ancient texts explain, if wind enters the body and depletes the breath, then a person's essence (Jing) is lost, and evil influences will injure the Liver.

Fire is associated with life in all its passion and vitality. In the cycle of birth, growth, and decay, fire is warm and nourishing, keeping life moving forward. When there is deficient fire, you cannot give or receive warmth in your life. Your life spark is dimmed. This may result in hot, painful joints, as if fire were stuck. Fevers may flare up and circulation may become poor, making some parts of the body cold, while others are hot. Varicose veins and digestive problems are possible results.

The Organ Systems that are aligned with fire are the Small Intestine, the Heart, the Triple Burner and Circulation Sex, which corresponds to the Pericardium in TCM.

The Small Intestine, paired with the Heart, separates the pure from the impure, physiologically, emotionally, and spiritually. Xue is affected by excess or deficient fire and the blood vessels are associated with fire as well. Furthermore, since the Heart is home to the spirit path or gate, where Shen resides, people who have fire as the dominant phase are usually charismatic, open-minded and empathetic. They seek similarities between people instead of differences. But if Heart becomes too dominant, a person may become easily confused, uncertain and oversensitive. A person may become afraid of not knowing where or who he or she is. In cases of extreme disharmony, the person becomes disturbed, even psychotic. When fire is unbalanced, the Shen is wounded, and joy, the emotion associated with fire, is lost or destroyed.

Circulation Sex is paired with the Triple Burner and has a powerful effect on the psyche. According to the Five Phases, Circulation Sex is associated with the vascular system and the circulation of fluids. The organ has no specific location. In Five Phases, the Triple Burner is associated with temperature maintenance and regulation. It impacts family relationships and social ties, plus sympathy and antipathy.

Metal represents functions that are declining. Metal is involved in the communication networks in the body that allow the intake of air and fuel and assimilate them into energy. A deficiency of metal causes a breakdown in the mind/body/spirit.

The Lung System is associated with metal and an imbalance in metal is associated with asthma, bronchitis, or emphysema. The Lung System also fuels emotions (overwhelming beauty is said to be breathtaking) and a metal imbalance can produce grief and deep sadness. A person who is Lung dominant is said to be ethereal, creative, intuitive, even psychic. When Lung becomes overly dominant, the emotions may veer out of control, and the person may have difficulty dealing with change and may swing between being a passive victim and a tyrannical dictator.

The Large Intestine is associated with metal. Its function is to remove waste from the body. Any imbalance of metal may make it difficult for the body to rid itself of toxic substances and emotions.

Water takes the shape of whatever contains it and can be hot, cold, liquid, solid, clear, or murky. In the body water enlivens every cell and the blood, tears, urine, sweat and other liquids.

The Kidney System is associated with water. It is the storehouse of what is called the vital essences and acts as the gateway to the stomach. A person who is Kidney dominant is often a visionary, imaging future possibilities and seeing his or her own destiny clearly. If knocked down, this person gets right back up and fights again. However, if the Kidney becomes too dominant, the person may slide into suspiciousness, fear of getting close to others and a sense of separation or falling apart. When the Kidney System is in disharmony, the Shen is volatile. You may feel like you are drowning in your fears. Physically, Kidney-dominant people may experience lethargy, edema, urination, and back problems. It is also associated with hypertension.

Earth denotes balance. Healthy earth provides a feeling of contentedness and purpose. When it is unbalanced, disruption of basic cycles of sleep, menstruation, appetite, breathing, and fertility may occur.

Earth's role as the center is revealed in its association with the Spleen System, which is the source of life for all other Organ Systems. It is also aligned with the Stomach, which influences formation of ideas and opinions. Those who are earth dominant are characterized as reliable, sedate, nurturing, and supportive. They have excellent memory for details and like to be the center of things. When earth becomes dominant, they can become obsessive, they may drown in their own mental contents, and they may lose the ability to associate ideas logically. Physically, they may experience trouble with digestion and absorption of food.

IDENTIFYING YOUR FIVE PHASES CHARACTERISTICS

Q: Would you characterize yourself as
    a. Ethereal and creative
    b. Open-minded and empathetic
    c. Able to imagine your destiny clearly
    d. Reliable and nurturing
    e. A take-charge kind of person

A: If you answered A, you may have a constitution characteristic of metal.
If you said B, fire. If you said C, water. If you said D, earth. If you said E, wood.

Q: Which emotion do you feel is strongest in you? Anger, meditation/concentration, fear, sadness or joy?

A: Anger is associated with wood, meditation/concentration with earth, fear with water, sadness with metal, joy with fire.

FIVE PHASES ASSOCIATIONS

	Wood	*Fire*	*Earth*	*Metal*	*Water*
Transitions	Birth	Growth	Transformation	Harvest	Storing
Direction	East	South	Center	West	North
Color	Green	Red	Yellow	White	Black
Climate	Wind	Heat	Damp	Dry	Cold
Human sound	Shout	Laugh	Sing	Weep	Groan
Emotion	Anger	Joy	Meditation	Grief/sadness	Fright/fear
Taste	Sour	Bitter	Sweet	Pungent	Salty
Yin organ	Liver	Heart/pericardium	Spleen	Lung	Kidney
Yang organ	Gallbladder	Small Intestine Triple Burner	Stomach	Large Intestine	Bladder
Sense organ	Eye	Tongue	Mouth	Nose	Ear
Tissue	Tendons	Blood	Muscle	Skin and hair	Bones
Smell	Goatish	Burning	Fragrant	Putrid	Rotten
Grains	Wheat	Corn	Millet	Rice	Beans
Season	Spring	Summer	Late summer and change of seasons	Fall	Winter

CHAPTER THREE

Roots of Disharmony

Causes of Disease in Chinese Medicine

Ancient Chinese medicine does not talk about viruses or bacteria as triggers of disease or disorders. Instead, it talks about influences that cause disharmony in Yin/Yang, the Essential Substances, the Organ Systems, the channels and the Five Phases.

There are several categories of influences that produce disharmony: The Six Pernicious Influences and the Seven Emotions are the two main ones.

THE SIX PERNICIOUS INFLUENCES

The Six Pernicious Influences—Heat, Cold, Wind, Dampness, Dryness and Summer Heat—are external climatic forces that can invade the body and create disharmony in the mind/body/spirit. For example, if you are exposed to Excess Heat or Cold or Wind for a long time, or if you are exposed to the influences when your body is already weak, you may develop an illness. This illness, triggered by external influences, can migrate inward and become more serious—as a slight cold might become pneumonia. This happens when the External Pernicious Influences overpower the body's natural protection against disease.

COLD

When hypothermia hits a skier or a mountain climber, muscle control fades, motion becomes slow and awkward, fatigue sets in and the body shuts down. That's the same effect that the Cold Pernicious Influence has. It saps the body's energy and makes movements cumbersome. The tongue becomes pale; the pulse is slow. A person may develop a fear of cold and feel like sleeping in a curled-up position. Cold is Yin, and when it invades the body, it chills all or part of it. If there's pain, it's eased by warmth.

When External Cold attacks the body, acute illness may develop, along with chills, fever and body aches. When the External Cold moves inward and becomes an interior disharmony, it is associated with a chronic condition that produces a pale face, lethargy and grogginess, a craving for heat and a tendency to sleep for longer than usual periods of time.

HEAT

Heat disorders feel like you've been playing tennis for two hours in the blazing sun. You're weary and at the same time, strangely cranked up. You can't stop talking about the game, but your words stick in your mouth. You don't feel like yourself again until you cool down and quench your thirst.

Heat disorders cause overactive Yang functions or insufficient Yin functions. They are generally associated with bodily heat, a red face, hyperactivity and talkativeness, fever, thirst for cold liquids and a rapid pulse. Symptoms include carbuncles and boils, dry mouth and thirst. Confused speech and delirium arise when heat attacks the Shen.

DAMPNESS

Think about what happens to your backyard when it rains for two days. It becomes soggy and water collects in stagnant pools. That is how Dampness affects the body. Damp pain is heavy and expansive. Dampness blocks the flow of life energy and causes a stuffy chest and abdomen.

When External Dampness invades, it enters the Channels and causes stiff joints and heavy limbs. When Dampness invades the Spleen, it can cause upset stomach, nausea, lack of appetite, a swollen abdomen and diarrhea.

Interior Dampness—caused by either the penetration of External Dampness to the Interior or by a breakdown in the Spleen's transformation of fluids—is associated with mucus, which in Chinese medicine is more than simply bodily secretions. It is produced when the Spleen or Kidney is beset with disharmony and can cause obstructions and produce tumors, coughing, and if it invades the Shen, can lead to erratic behavior and insanity. Once Dampness has taken root, it is hard to displace.

DRYNESS

Dryness is a frequent partner with Heat; just think about the cracked bottom of a dried-up riverbed. Heat creates redness and warmth, and Dryness creates evaporation and dehydration. External Dryness invading the body may create respiratory problems such as asthmatic breathing and a dry cough, acute pain and fever.

SUMMER HEAT

This Pernicious Influence feels like the humid, oppressive weather that creates the dog days of August. It attacks the body after exposure to extreme heat and causes a sudden high fever and total lethargy. It is always an external influence and often arises along with dampness.

WIND

Wind animates the body, stirring it from repose into motion just as wind moves the leaves of a tree. When Wind enters the body, it is usually joined to another influence such as Cold.

If the body is infiltrated by Wind, the first symptoms usually appear on the skin, in the lungs, or on the face. Tics, twitches, fear of drafts, headaches and a stuffed-up nose are symptoms.

When External Wind invades the body more deeply, it can cause seizures, ringing in the ears and dizziness.

STAGES OF HEAT- AND COLD-INDUCED PATTERNS OF DISHARMONY

When Heat or Cold invade the body, they create stages of disharmony. The symptoms associated with these stages help in the process of diagnosis and treatment. (Remember, Chinese medicine is not linear. These six stages can appear in any order and some may not appear at all.) When a Cold-induced disharmony moves into the body, it may pass in some order through one or more of the following six stages.

1. Taiyang (*tie-yang*) is characterized by cold, fever, headache, a stiff neck, and what is called a floating pulse. (The discussion of pulses follows on page 73.)
2. Yangming (*yang-ming*) is characterized by fever, no fear of cold/aversion to heat, irritability, thirst, possible digestive symptoms such as fullness and constipation and a full pulse. This is a stage of Interior Heat disharmony because Cold induces heat in both the first and second stages.
3. Shaoyang (*shau-yang*) is characterized by malaria-like alteration of cold and fever, no appetite, a bitter taste in the mouth, tenderness along the sides, the urge to vomit and a wiry pulse.
4. Taiyin (*tie-yin*) is characterized by vomiting, loss of appetite, pain and diarrhea but no thirst. This is associated with a Deficient Spleen System.
5. Shaoyin (*shau-yin*) is characterized by profound sleepiness, cold and a weak

pulse. Fever disappears. This is associated with deficient Yang of the Kidney System. Rarely, it causes a Yin-deficient hot condition.

6. Jueyin (*zh-way-yin*) is characterized by upper-body heat and lower-body cold together.

When a Heat-induced disharmony moves into the body, it may pass in some order through one or more of the following four stages:

1. **The Wei** (*way*) stage. The body's natural defenses are attacked, and the result may be fever, slight fear of cold, coughing, headache, a reddish tongue and a quick floating pulse.

2. **The Qi** (*chee*) stage. The Pernicious Influence penetrates the protective defenses of the body. The main symptom is usually high fever without chills, but symptoms vary, depending on which Organ System is affected. For example, Heat in the Lung produces high fever and coughing, while Heat in the Stomach produces high fever, abdominal pain and constipation.

3. **The Ying** (*ying*) stage. Deeper penetration by pernicious Heat increases the disharmony in mind/body/spirit. The symptoms of this stage include a bright red tongue, an easily disturbed spirit, restlessness and even mania, a rapid pulse, dark yellow urine, less thirstiness than in the Qi stage and possible skin eruptions.

4. **Xue** (*sch-whey*) stage. In the fourth and deepest stage, the Pernicious Influence of Heat enters the blood, exacerbating third-stage symptoms. Severe rashes, skin eruptions, high fever and even coma may result. Blood in urine or vomit may appear. Heat can injure the Yin, producing symptoms such as low fever, hot palms, dry teeth, a thin pulse and stiffness and unresponsiveness.

EPIDEMIC FACTORS

In addition to the Six Pernicious Influences there are also infectious Epidemic Factors. They trigger symptoms that are similar to the Pernicious Influence Heat, but are severely toxic and cause the sudden onset of diseases such as cholera and plague. Some diseases—particularly viral diseases such as HIV—that do not always have an apparent sudden onset are also triggered by Epidemic Factors. Most of these factors fit into a category called Heat Toxin.

THE SEVEN EMOTIONS

While the Six Pernicious Influences are generally external triggers of disharmony, the Seven Emotions are internal causes of disease.

THE SEVEN EMOTIONS

- Joy
- Anger
- Fear and Fright
- Sadness
- Grief and Meditation

These emotions are as real a source of disharmony in the mind/body/spirit as the External Pernicious Influences. In Chinese medicine, a disease is never dismissed as being all in your head. Chinese medicine does not divide diseases or disorders into neat little packages—this one physical, that one emotional, this one psychological, that one spiritual. Chinese medicine views the human being as a whole. There is no separation between the body and the emotions, between the body and the spirit, or between the body and the forces that shape the quality of daily life.

However, despite this recognition of the importance of the Seven Emotions in diagnosing disharmony, Traditional Chinese Medicine, as developed and practiced in postrevolutionary China, does not place as large an emphasis on the Seven Emotions as it does on the Pernicious Influences. On the other hand, the Five Phases system pays special attention to emotions and offers the TCM practitioner useful insights when diagnosing emotion-based disharmonies.

DISHARMONIES OF THE SEVEN EMOTIONS

An Excess or Deficiency of any emotion is indicative of disharmony in the mind and spirit, and it alerts the Chinese medicine practitioner to disharmonies in Organ Systems as well. The Heart and Liver are the most susceptible to emotions. The Heart stores the Shen and unharmonious emotions can disturb the Shen and cause sleeplessness, muddled thinking, inappropriate crying or laughing, and in extreme cases, fits, madness and hysteria. Excess or deficient joy especially impacts the Heart. The Liver, which is responsible for the movement of energy, Xue and emotions, is associated with anger. If the Liver energy is stuck or in disharmony, the emotions become suppressed. If the emotions become suppressed, they suppress the function of the Liver. Sadness and grief, which are associated but distinct states, take their toll on the Lungs. Too much or too little meditation will cause the Spleen to become unbalanced. Fear, which is a sustained, inner emotion, and fright, which is a reactive, more external emotion, interfere with the smooth functioning of the Kidney.

OTHER SOURCES OF DISHARMONY

POOR NUTRITION

A balanced diet is an essential component of good health, and in Chinese medicine, it is used as a powerful therapeutic tool. The Chinese system recognizes that diet exerts a strong influence over the mind/body/spirit. Digestive problems, depletion of energy, depression and many specific disharmonies can be triggered by eating too much or too little, by eating too frequently or not often enough, by eating food that is too cold or by eating too many raw foods and by eating food that is impure or unsanitary. This happens, in part, because the Stomach and Spleen Systems, which receive and transform food, are the most sensitive to diet. When they become imbalanced, many associated components of the mind/body/spirit are affected.

Harmony can be restored by eating a diet that helps counter the disharmonies. For example, if you are suffering from Interior Cold Deficiency, then your practitioner may suggest you eat foods that are warming and sweet, to help rebuild your Qi. For more information on how diet can counter disharmonies see chapter 6 and 7.

UNHARMONIOUS SEX

Excessive sex can cause deficiency disorders, especially in men.

EXCESS PHYSICAL ACTIVITY

Obsessive exercise, overworking, and high-stress situations all deplete the mind/body/spirit and make the body vulnerable to disharmony and disease.

CHAPTER FOUR

Disharmony Revealed

The Eight Fundamental Patterns and the Pathology of Essential Substances, Organ Systems and Channels

In Chinese medicine texts, there is no discussion of diseases or disorders as we know them in the West. You don't catch the flu; you develop a disharmony.

In the beginning, that may make it difficult to understand how your Chinese medicine practitioner describes what ails you. For example, you go for help because you have migraines; the practitioner may offer to treat you for disharmonies such as Stagnant Liver Qi, Liver Heat, Dampness, Deficient Qi and Xue or Excess Yang, depending on the signs and symptoms that accompany your headache. The headache is viewed as a symptom, not the underlying disorder, which requires treatment.

To help clarify the difference between Chinese and Western concepts of illness and disharmony this chapter outlines the Eight Fundamental Patterns of disharmony and details how Chinese medicine describes disturbances in Organ Systems channels and Essential Substances.

WESTERN DISEASES AND ASSOCIATED TCM DISHARMONIES

In Chinese medicine, the diagnosis of a disharmony is highly individualized: Two people with the same Western ailment may not have the same disharmony. A disharmony, unlike a disease, is not defined only by its physical manifestations but also by how it influences the harmony of the Essential Substances, the Organ Systems and the mind/body/spirit as a whole.

EXAMPLES OF WESTERN DISEASES AND SYNDROMES AND ASSOCIATED TRADITIONAL CHINESE MEDICINE PATTERNS OF DISHARMONY

Western Diagnosis	Possible TCM Patterns
Alcoholism	Shen disturbance Liver Damp-Heat Spleen Qi Deficiency Liver Qi Stagnation Liver Fire Dampness
Cervical dysplasia	**Heat toxin with:** Yin Deficiency in Liver and Kidney Damp-Heat in the Liver channel associated with Spleen Qi Deficiency
Common Cold	Wind-Heat Wind-Cold Taiyang stage Cold disease Qi stage Hot disease
Depression	Shen disturbance Liver Fire Liver Qi Stagnation Heart Xue Deficiency
Essential hypertension	Liver Yang Rising Kidney Deficiency Essential hypertension Qi and Xue Deficiency Yin Deficiency/Yang Excess
Food poisoning	Summer Heat Food Stagnation in Stomach
Hepatitis	Liver/Gallbladder Damp-Heat Spleen Damp-Cold Spleen Deficiency Xue Deficiency Spleen Damp-Heat Qi Stagnation Qi Deficiency Xue Stagnation
Irritable bowel syndrome	Spleen Qi Deficiency Large Intestine Dryness Spleen Yang Deficiency Large Intestine Heat Spleen Qi Deficiency with Dampness Liver Qi Stagnation Large Intestine Damp Heat

Menopausal syndrome	Deficient Kidney Yin
	Deficient Kidney Yang
	Deficient Liver Xue
	Deficient Kidney Yin and Yang
Migraine	Qi and Xue Deficiency
	Liver Heat
	Dampness
	Liver Qi Stagnation
	Deficient Yin/Excess Yang
	Stomach Heat
PMS	**Liver Qi Stagnation with:**
	Heart Xue Deficiency
	Liver Xue Deficiency
	Depressive Liver Fire
	Spleen Qi Deficiency
	Stomach Heat
	Dampness
Sinusitis	Wind-Damp
	Wind-Damp-Heat
	Wind-Damp-Cold
	Lung Phlegm-Heat

THE EIGHT FUNDAMENTAL PATTERNS

The Eight Fundamental Patterns, which are paired as Interior, Exterior; Heat, Cold; Excess, Deficiency; and Yin, Yang, describe the way in which the Pernicious Influences and Seven Emotions create disharmony in the mind/body/spirit. They also reveal the dynamic association of complementary yet opposed forces (Yin/Yang) within the body that have been thrown off balance by the presence of an influence or other disharmony.

Interior and Exterior patterns tell the practitioner where in the body the disease resides.

Interior patterns of disharmony are indicated if the disharmony is chronic, produces changes in urine and stool, if there is discomfort or pain in the torso and if there is no aversion to cold or wind.

Exterior patterns of disharmony often come on suddenly and are acute. Common signs include chills, fever, a dislike of cold and an achy feeling overall.

Heat and Cold describe the activity of the body and the nature of the disease. Cold patterns are caused by Deficient Yang or an External Cold Pernicious Influence. With Cold everything slows down, a person becomes withdrawn, and sleeps in a curled-up position. Pain is relieved by warmth; bodily secretions are thin and clear; and there is a desire for warm liquids.

Heat patterns are caused by invasion of External Heat Pernicious Influence, the depletion of Yin substances, and Excess Yang. With Heat, the body's processes speed up and a person may talk excessively, have a red face and hot body, and prefer cold beverages; secretions become thick, putrid, and dark.

Deficiency and excess express the impact of the disharmony on the body's resistance to disease (Normal Qi). With Deficiency, there is underactivity in the Organ System(s), weakness and tentative movement, a pale or ashen face, sweating, incontinence, shallow breathing, and pain that is relieved by pressure. Excess is associated with overactivity of bodily functions; heavy, forceful movements; a loud, full voice; heavy breathing; and pain increased by pressure.

BODY SIGNS

Learning to "read" your body and to associate what you observe with Chinese medicine's way of describing balance and imbalance will enhance your ability to harmonize your mind/body/spirit.

Take a minute to think over your medical history. Have you ever had an illness that you could identify as Excess? As Deficient? Can you recall having an illness that made you have an aversion to the cold? How about one in which cold did not bother you?

Yin and Yang encompass the other six Fundamental Patterns. Yin encompasses Interior, Cold, and Deficient; Yang encompasses Exterior, Heat, and Excess.

To determine Yin/Yang disharmony, the doctor searches for clues about whether the disharmony is interior or exterior; clues about patterns of Heat and Cold; and clues about patterns of Deficiency and Excess. These can be translated into clinical symptoms. Patterns of Heat and Excess, for example, show themselves in fast, forceful movements and by pain that is intensified by pressure and soothed by cold. If these qualities are observed, the doctor will then know that there is a Heat Excess Yang condition. (For detailed information about the diagnostic process, see chapter 5.)

After examining the influence of the Eight Pernicious Influences and the Seven Emotions and the patterns of disharmony, the next step is to explore the pathologies of the Essential Substances, Organ Systems and channels. This will demonstrate how the influences lead to disharmony, the many ways that disharmonies can manifest themselves and what disharmonies do to the balance of the mind/body/spirit.

THE PATHOLOGY OF THE ESSENTIAL SUBSTANCES: QI, SHEN, XUE, JING AND JIN-YE

QI DISHARMONIES

When Qi moves harmoniously throughout the body, there is wholeness and good health. When it is disrupted, disharmony and illness can arise. Unbalanced Qi may become Deficient or Excess.

Excess Qi almost always collects and pools and becomes Stagnant. Excess and Stagnant Qi are associated with blockages in the channels and Organ Systems that interfere with the circulation of Qi and cause it to pool up, depriving some areas of the body and flooding others. The blockages may occur because of suppressed emotions, Pernicious Influences, poor diet, or traumatic injury. The symptoms of Excess and Stagnant Qi are pain that worsens with pressure and is not easy to pinpoint, a feeling of overall fullness, and belching that may relieve the pain. You may ache all over and have trouble sitting still. Often the pain waxes and wanes and is related to your emotional state.

When Stagnant Qi becomes more severe, it may actually reverse direction and become *Rebellious.* This disharmony causes vomiting, belching, hiccups, coughing, asthma, liver disturbances and fainting.

Deficient Qi occurs when bad diet, lack of exercise, respiration problems, and/ or disharmony of the spirit and mind use up Qi and don't replenish it. It can trigger spontaneous sweating, fatigue, weakness, lack of a desire to move, a weak voice, a pale but bright face, disharmony of a particular organ system and symptoms that become worse when you exert yourself. Deficient Qi is relatively Yin.

If the condition worsens, Deficient Qi may become *Sinking or Collapsed Qi.* Sinking Qi is associated with prolapse of an organ (when it sags or falls down, such as a prolapsed uterus or bladder), dizziness, lack of stamina, and a bright, pale face.

SHEN DISHARMONIES

Shen disharmonies usually are triggered by internal emotional disharmonies (an imbalance of one of the Seven Emotions) and are often accompanied by Stagnant Qi (depression) and disharmony of the Heart and Liver Systems. If there is Deficient Heart Xue leading to Shen disturbance, there may also be an underlying Deficient Spleen condition.

Disturbed Shen causes forgetfulness, disorientation, memory lapses, insomnia, and lackluster eyes. Extreme disharmony is associated with madness.

Lack of Shen is associated with a flat affect and inability to communicate. The classic phrase, "The lights are on, but no one's home," describes this state.

To a Chinese medicine doctor, it makes no sense to heal the corporal body without healing the Shen (or spirit) because the physical and spiritual are inseparable parts of the human being. Disharmony in the Shen is often the first hint of developing disharmonies and disease. Feeling out of sorts, fatigued, blue, grumpy and dispirited may indicate that an illness is developing. If the practitioner and the client intercede early, when the Shen is only mildly unbalanced, the development of full-blown disorders and disease may be forestalled.

XUE DISHARMONIES

Deficient Xue is associated with malnutrition, loss of blood, Spleen Deficiency, depletion of Qi, and emotional stress. It can trigger insomnia, dry skin, dizziness, hair loss, palpitations, menstrual irregularities, and blurry vision. When Xue is Deficient, the body doesn't receive sufficient nourishment, often in one or more Organ Systems. When the whole body is Deficient in Xue, the skin has a pallor and is dry.

   Excess or Stagnant Xue is either caused by direct damage to the body's tissues (i.e., falling while skating) or is a result of Stagnant Qi, Deficient Xue and Cold Obstructing Xue. Symptoms include sharp, stabbing, fixed pain, tumors, or swollen organs. Only in pregnancy may an increase in Xue and fluids be healthy and not associated with an Excess disharmony.

JING DISHARMONIES

We are born with Jing, and can either deplete or replenish it throughout our lives. It always tends toward deficiency. *Deficient Jing* symptoms include congenital disabilities, improper maturation, premature aging, sexual problems and infertility. Disharmony of Jing is associated with Deficient Kidney.

JIN-YE DISHARMONIES

Jin-Ye may be either Deficient or Excess. *Deficient Jin-Ye* is associated with dry lips, hair, eyes, and skin. *Excess Jin-Ye* causes stagnation of fluids and produces edema and swelling.

THE EFFECT OF DISHARMONY ON THE ORGAN SYSTEMS

When external and internal Pernicious Influences create disharmony, they upset the balance within and between each Organ System and the various channels. Each Organ System has its own patterns of disharmony and associated symptoms.

THE ZANG (YIN) ORGAN SYSTEMS

Kidney System

When the Kidney System becomes imbalanced, it may have one of four patterns of disharmony: Deficient Yang, Deficient Qi, Deficient Yin and Deficient Jing. Such disruptions are often associated with the emotional state of fear and with the exercise of (or lack of ability to exercise) the will.

Deficient Kidney System is associated with impotence, hearing loss and incontinence. It is often associated with cold limbs; lack of Shen; swollen limbs; profuse, clear urine; sore lower back; and loose teeth.

Deficient Kidney System Qi may trigger frequent urination, incontinence, bed-wetting, asthmatic breathing and low back pain.

Deficient Kidney System Yin is associated with hot palms and soles, dry mouth, thirst, constipation, red cheeks, afternoon fevers, night sweats, insomnia, ringing in the ears, premature ejaculation, forgetfulness, and low back pain.

Deficient Kidney System Jing may lead to infertility, premature aging, retarded growth, lack or retardation of initial menstrual periods and stiff joints.

> A thirty-three-year-old woman, who was unable to become pregnant, came to the clinic after having been given progestin and Clomid, which made her ill. She hadn't had her period for six years—since going off birth control pills. As a teenager, she had painful periods associated with vomiting. She said she was cold most of the time.
>
> She was diagnosed with Deficient Kidney Qi and treated with Korean constitutional acupuncture, moxibustion, and herbs.
>
> After several treatments, she reported she felt warmer, and after two months, her pulse changed from slow, which is associated with Cold, to wiry, which is associated with Stagnant Qi. She became angry and depressed for a while, as her body went through a series of adjustments. We then had to change the treatment to regulate the Qi. At the same time, she started ovulating and began to have regular menstrual periods.
>
> Twelve months after beginning treatment, she became pregnant. She now has a healthy four-year-old and a one-year-old.

Spleen System

Spleen System disharmony in general manifests itself in loose stools, abdominal fullness and distention, nausea and poor appetite. Anxiety and the inability to concentrate are also associated with Spleen System imbalance. Interior Spleen disharmonies are caused by congenital weakness, malnutrition, or chronic diseases and excessive mental activity.

Deficient Spleen System Qi symptoms are loose stools, poor appetite, abdominal distention and pain, pale complexion, fatigue and lethargy, weight gain due to fluid retention, edema, shortness of breath and a pale, bright face. A subset of Deficient Spleen Qi is *Sinking Spleen System Qi*, characterized by muscular weakness and prolapsed organs, particularly of the uterus, bladder, and rectum. *Spleen System Not Able to Govern the Xue*, another subset of Deficient Spleen Qi, is associated with Xue circulating outside its proper pathways. The symptoms are chronic bleeding such as bloody stools, nosebleeds, varicose veins, hemorrhoids, excessive menstrual bleeding, nonmenstrual uterine bleeding, easy bruising and purpura (purple spotting indicative of bleeding beneath the skin).

One of the most persistent cases of Deficient Spleen Qi leading to Spleen Not Being Able to Govern Xue was that of a young woman in her thirties who had gone to a Western doctor for spotting between periods, easy bruising, excessively heavy periods, fatigue and abdominal distention. The Western doctor hadn't been able to solve the problems.

I recommended she switch to a diet with no raw foods and use moxibustion on certain acupuncture points to help bleeding and eradicate the pain of the varicose veins. After six weeks, the spotting had stopped and her energy returned.

Deficient Spleen System Qi Leading to Dampness is a deficiency condition leading to excess. (See excess syndromes below.)

Deficient Spleen System Qi Leading to Spleen Not Being Able to Govern the Xue is associated with spotting between periods, internal bleeding, easy bruising and varicose veins.

Deficient Spleen System Yang develops from chronic Deficient Spleen Qi and Cold. The symptoms are the same as for Deficient Spleen Qi, plus clear, copious urine, cold extremities and body, edema, weak digestion and the desire for hot beverages.

Deficient Spleen System Yin appears in end-stage, life-threatening illnesses, such as AIDS and diabetes (without the benefit of insulin). The symptoms include severe dryness, especially of the skin and lips, unquenchable thirst, loss of lean muscle mass and severe wasting. Fever appears every afternoon and often in the evenings.

Externally caused Excess Spleen System patterns are often a result of an underlying Deficient Spleen condition. They include Damp/Cold and Damp/Heat.

Damp/Cold occurs when Spleen Yang becomes trapped by exposure to excessive Dampness. This can happen if you are being drenched by rain, wade through cold water, or are exposed to cold/damp temperatures for a prolonged time. The associated symptoms are lack of appetite, watery stools, a lusterless, yellow face, fatigue, and no thirst.

Damp/Heat occurs when External Dampness and Heat invade the body or when Spleen System Qi leads to Excess Damp and combines with Heat. It results in the slowing of bodily functions, causing an accumulation of fluids. The symptoms are lack of appetite, a feeling of fullness in the stomach, scanty, dark urine and fatigue. Sometimes it is associated with thirst without the desire to drink, itchy skin and fever. It may also be associated with acute viral hepatitis.

Liver System

Repression of emotions is the most frequent cause of Liver problems, which can manifest themselves in various patterns.

Stagnant Liver System Qi is the most common and the first Liver disorder to appear when the system becomes imbalanced. It is an Excess condition and relatively Yang. The causes of Liver Qi Stagnation are emotional suppression and trauma. This leads to depression, uncomfortable feelings, discomfort and pain between the ribs and in the chest, breast, and diaphragm, abdominal distention, restlessness, premenstrual congestion or distention, and a quick temper.

Stagnant Liver System Xue is characterized by fixed, sharp, stabbing pains and palpable masses. It often develops from Stagnant Liver Qi. In women, it is associated with missed menstrual periods, menstrual clotting and cramps, or severe trauma. In men, this pattern's appearance is almost always the result of severe trauma or severe illness.

Liver System Yang (or Fire) Rising develops when Stagnant Liver System Qi becomes more congested and severe. It is associated with an accumulation of Heat, and symptoms include headaches; eye pain; red eyes; sharp chest pain; scanty, yellow urine; vertigo; nosebleeds; fits of anger; and dry stools. If left unchecked, this pattern can develop into a more serious condition—*Interior Liver System Wind*—which is associated with strokes, high fever with convulsions, paralysis and loss of consciousness.

> A woman, thirty-eight, in the first month of pregnancy, came for treatment of severe nausea that lasted all day and was uncontrolled by ingestion of food. The symptoms were clear signs of Liver Qi Stagnation. In addition, she was an enthusiastic jogger and used it to control stress, but she was unable to continue running and this only increased her disharmony.
>
> She was put on a program of diet therapy and acupuncture. She had to eliminate chicken and turkey for the duration of the pregnancy since they congest Liver Qi and cause stagnation. She also received one acupuncture treatment and short-term herbs. Within two days, the nausea stopped. A month later, when she tried to eat chicken, her nausea returned briefly.

Deficient Liver System Xue is characterized by general Dryness without any Heat symptoms. The symptoms are dryness of the eyes and nails, blurry vision, dizziness, muscle spasms, reduced menstrual periods, twitching and a pale, lusterless face.

Deficient Liver System Yin includes all the symptoms of Deficient Liver Xue, plus red cheeks and eyes, restlessness, hot flashes, headaches, dizziness, numb limbs, night sweats, dry mouth and throat, ringing in the ears and a quick temper.

Damp-heat of Liver System can occur when the diet is of poor quality and food is heavily spiced and fatty. The symptoms are discomfort in the top of the shoulders and rib cage, a bitter taste in the mouth, poor appetite, scanty, dark urine, jaundice, fever and chills. Damp-heat of the Liver System is associated with hepatitis and inflammation of the Gallbladder.

Cold Obstructing the Liver System Channel tends to be a male disharmony. Symptoms include a swollen scrotum and distention in the groin, which is relieved by warmth.

Deficient Liver System Qi is quite rare. It creates Deficient Qi in the whole body, leading to a breakdown in joint function, general lethargy, shallow breathing, a lack of forcefulness in voice and spontaneous sweating.

Lung System

General symptoms of Lung System disharmonies include dry skin or skin eruptions, shortness of breath on exertion, cough, asthma, allergies, nose and throat disorders, low resistance to Exterior Pernicious Influences and reduced energy. Grief and the ability to let go at the proper time are also associated with the Lung System. There are also symptoms associated with specfic types of Lung System disharmony.

Patterns of Exterior Excess Lung System Disharmonies include the following.

Wind Cold, which is associated with chills, head and body aches, frothy, thin, clear or white phlegm, and a lack of sweating;

Wind Heat, which is associated with fever, slight chills, sore throat, some sweating, a coarse cough, and thick, yellow sticky phlegm;

Wind Dryness, which is associated with a fever with chills, headache, dry throat and nose, and scant, dry phlegm.

Patterns of Interior Excess Lung System Disharmonies include the following.

Dampness, which is generally triggered by a pre-existing lack of Spleen and Kidney function. It is associated with a full, high-pitched cough, chest inflammation, difficulty breathing when lying down, wheezing, copious phlegm, no thirst and a swollen face.

Heat is generally triggered by overactive Liver and Heart Systems or the penetration of an External Pernicious Influence. When it is caused by the Liver invading the Lungs, the symptoms are dryness, pain in the chest or ribs, chest distention and choking cough with thick, green phlegm. When it's caused by the Heart System, the symptoms are insomnia, restlessness, cough, agitation and confusion. When caused by an Exterior Pernicious Influence, the symptoms are fever, sweating, cough, shortness of breath and a rapid, superficial pulse.

Deficient Lung System patterns include the following.

Deficient Lung System Qi, which appears when the External Excess Pernicious Influence remains in the Lung and injures the Qi or when there are other Interior disharmonies that affect the Lungs. The symptoms are a whispering voice, reluctance to speak, weak respiration, susceptibility to colds, weak cough, spontaneous sweating, shortness of breath that is worse with exertion, lack of warmth and thin, white phlegm.

A thirty-five-year-old man, who had asthma since he was a child, came to the clinic after a bout of mononucleosis, which had lowered his resistance to pollens and molds. He was fatigued, his asthma had become so severe that he'd had to give up regular exercise, and he was using two kinds of inhalers constantly. He was coughing up white phlegm, was short of breath, and quite lethargic.

He was diagnosed as Deficient Lung Qi with Dampness due to Deficient Spleen. His treatment included acupuncture and moxibustion to the Lung System points on the upper back along with other tonification points. For acute asthma attacks, he was prescribed herbal pills to use as needed. For the underlying deficiency, he was given a constitutional herbal formula.

"After a few months, I noticed that the herbs had reduced the phlegm and I was able to wean myself off the inhalers," the man said. "During the last allergy season, which was a pretty intense one, I did great."

Deficient Lung System Yin is associated with Deficienᵗ Fluids of the Lung. The causes are Internal Dryness, chronic Deficient Kidney Yin, and the external Pernicious Influence of Heat remaining in the lung and causing dryness. Symptoms are fatigue, weakness, dry cough with no phlegm, restlessness, insomnia, afternoon fevers, night sweats, dry mouth and throat, weak voice, red cheeks, varicose veins, a feverish sensation in the palms, soles, and chest (Five Centers Heat), and sometimes scanty phlegm, streaked with blood.

BODY SIGNS

Have you ever experienced Deficient Spleen System Qi—fatigue, lethargy, abdominal distention, fluid retention, pale complexion? Or Excess Lung System wind-cold—chills, head and body aches, clear or white phlegm, and lack of sweating? In Western medicine these symptoms, respectively, may be identified as irritable bowel syndrome and influenza.

Heart System

Patterns of deficiencies of the heart include the following.

Deficient Heart System Xue is often associated with Deficient Spleen Qi, as the Spleen is responsible for making the Xue. The symptoms include a pale, lusterless face, dizziness, anxiety, confusion, excessive crying or laughing and difficulty falling asleep.

Deficient Heart System Yin includes the symptoms of Deficient Heart Xue plus heat symptoms such as palpitations, agitation, insomnia, waking up during the night, warm palms and soles, emotional instability, increased dreams, poor memory, night sweats, and physical and emotional hypersensitivity. It is often associated with Deficient Kidney Yin.

Deficient Heart System Qi is associated with the physiological problems of circulation such as irregular pulse, arrythmia, shortness of breath, fatigue and heart failure. Symptoms become worse with exercise.

A sixty-eight-year-old man with congestive heart failure and arrythmia came into the clinic because his cardiologist had not been able to do anything to stabilize his irregular heartbeat or shortness of breath. He also had severe fatigue and swelling in the ankles. He was Diagnosed as having Deficient Heart Qi and started on a once-a-week program of acupuncture, moxibustion, and leg and foot massage to stabilize his heartbeat and reduce swelling. In addition, he was on crutches because he needed a hip replacement, which made his treatment more difficult—the constant pain and physical strain aggravated his Qi Deficiency.

After six months of therapy, the swelling has gone away and his Western doctor reports that there has been no further deterioration of his congestive heart problem.

Deficient Heart System Yang includes the symptoms of Deficient Heart Qi plus Cold symptoms such as pain and distention in the chest, cold limbs and/or coldness throughout the whole body, purplish lips, and a slower, weaker heartbeat. It often appears with Deficient Kidney Yang and Deficient Lung Qi.

A subset of Deficient Heart Yang is *Collapse of Yang*, in which Yin and Yang can separate and the person is near death. Symptoms include profuse sweating, extremely cold limbs, purple lips and confusion.

Patterns diagnosed as excess include the following.

Excess Heart System Fire is caused by extreme emotional excitement, sunstroke, or excess consumption of hot, pungent foods, drinks or herbs. Symptoms include insomnia, restlessness, red face, scanty, burning urine with blood, inflammation or soreness of the tongue and mouth, or thirst.

Excess Phlegm Obstructing Heart System or misting of the orifices may arise from Spleen Dampness or simply from a general internal lack of proper fluid circulation. The symptoms include Shen disharmony (due to excess phlegm), aberrations of consciousness, coma or semicoma (in Chinese medicine it's called "dumb like a wooden chicken"), excessive weeping or laughing, depression or dullness, mania, incoherent speech, muttering to oneself, drooling and predisposition to stroke. There are two types of phlegm: cold and hot. Excess Cold Phlegm symptoms are a withdrawn, inward manner, muttering, staring at walls and sudden blackouts. Excess Hot Phlegm symptoms include hyperactivity, agitation, aggression, incessant talking and violent lashing-out behavior.

Heart System Qi Stagnation is associated with stuffy chest and difficult breathing. If it is the result of Stagnant Phlegm, there are the same symptoms plus excess phlegm expectoration, abdominal fullness, nausea and vomiting.

Stagnant Heart System Xue is associated with angina and pectoral pain, and results from Deficient Heart Qi or Deficient Heart Yang. Symptoms include palpitations, shortness of breath, irregular pulse, fixed, stabbing pain and a purple face.

Pericardium System

There is only one major pattern associated with the Pericardium and it is not an independent pattern: *Excess Phlegm Obstructing Heart System* or misting of the orifices (see page 54).

THE FU (YANG) ORGAN SYSTEMS

Stomach System

The patterns of disharmony that may afflict the Stomach include the following.

Food Retention in Stomach System is due to irregular eating habits, overeating, or eating hard-to-digest foods. Retention blocks passage of Qi in the abdomen, triggering distention, fullness, and pain in the abdomen, foul belching, regurgitation, anorexia, vomiting and difficult bowel movements.

Retention of Fluid in Stomach System Due to Cold is associated with a constitutional deficiency of Stomach Qi, complicated by the invasion of the Exterior Pernicious Influence, Cold. Eating too much cold or raw food can also trigger this pattern. Symptoms include fullness and pain in the stomach relieved by warmth, reflux of clear fluid, or vomiting after eating. This pattern is associated with prolonged disease.

Hyperactivity of Fire in Stomach System (also called Stomach Heat) may arise from eating too many hot, fatty foods and from depression. The symptoms include burning and pain in the stomach, thirst for cold beverages, bleeding gums, and scant, yellow urine. It's often associated with stomach ulcers, excessive appetite, constipation, and mouth ulcers.

Deficient Stomach System Yin occurs when hyperactivity of Fire in the Stomach (see above) consumes the Stomach Yin or when Stomach fluid dries up because of persistent Heat due to a prolonged disease with fever. Symptoms include burning stomach pain, an empty, uncomfortable feeling in the stomach, hunger without appetite, dry heaves, hiccups, dry mouth and throat and constipation.

Triple Burner System

One theory of disharmonies in the Triple Burner identifies the Exterior Pernicious Influence of Damp Heat as the cause of disease.

Damp Heat in the Upper Burner Damp invades the body and stays in the muscles and upper body, damaging Spleen Qi. Symptoms include extreme dislike of cold, mild or no fever, feeling like there is a soft band around the head, heavy arms and legs, a feeling that an elephant is standing on your chest, lack of thirst, distended stomach, noisy bowels, loose stools, and lack of facial expression.

Damp Heat in the Middle Burner can arise from the External Pernicious Influences of Summer Heat and Damp. It can also occur when Damp Heat from the

Upper Burner sinks into the Middle Burner. Poor nutrition is also a trigger. Symptoms are similar to those for invasion of Damp and Heat in the Stomach and Spleen: heavy arms, legs, and trunk; full, distended chest and stomach; nausea; vomiting; anorexia; loose but difficult stools; dark urine; feeling thirsty with little desire to drink; plus fever that can't be felt at the first touch of the skin but that becomes evident after the skin is felt for a rather long time. In severe cases, the Shen is disturbed and mental abilities are affected.

Damp Heat in the Lower Burner affects the lower intestines and Urinary Bladder and is associated with difficulties with urination and elimination. Symptoms include constipation; a hard, distended lower abdomen; and thirstiness without much inclination to drink anything.

The Gallbladder System

The Gallbladder System doesn't manifest any organ patterns separately from Damp Heat of the Liver. The symptoms associated with that pattern include discomfort in the chest, a bitter taste in the mouth, poor appetite, scanty, dark urine, jaundice, fever, and chills. General Gallbladder dysfunction can cause anger and impulsiveness, an inability to make up your mind, and general weakness of character.

Small Intestine System

Pain Due to Disturbance of Small Intestine System Qi may result from poor nutrition, from carrying overly heavy loads, and/or wearing clothing that's inappropriate for the weather, which makes you vulnerable to External Pernicious Influences. Symptoms include acute lower abdominal pain, abdominal distention, noisy bowels and a heavy, downward-pushing sensation in the testes accompanied by lower back pain.

Heart Fire Moving to the Small Intestine System includes the symptoms of Heart Fire (see page 54) plus irritability; cold sores; sore throat; frequent, painful urination; and a full feeling in the lower abdomen.

Large Intestine System

Large Intestine System Damp Heat is sometimes called Damp Heat Dysentery. This pattern often occurs in hot climates in the summer and autumn when the Exterior Pernicious Influences of Summer Heat, Dampness and Toxic Heat invade the Stomach and the Intestines. It may also arise when a person eats too much raw or cold food, unsanitary food, or doesn't eat at regular times. The symptoms include abdominal pain, a feeling of urgency along with difficult bowel movements, watery diarrhea, bloody stools with mucus, burning anus and dark-colored urine. Sometimes it is accompanied with fever and thirst.

Consumption of Fluid of Large Intestine System is often seen in the elderly, after childbirth, and in the later stages of disease with fever. Symptoms include constipation, dry stools and dry mouth and throat.

Intestinal Abscess is known in Western medicine as appendicitis. The symptoms include acute pain in the lower right quadrant, aversion to touch and possibly a fever.

Urinary Bladder System

The main pattern of disharmony associated with the Bladder System is *Damp Heat in the Bladder System.* This pattern can arise from the invasion of Exterior Pernicious Dampness and Heat or from a diet of excessively hot, greasy, and sweet foods. Symptoms include painful, frequent, urgent urination; cloudy, dark urine; back pain; blood in urine; feeling of fullness in the lower abdomen; burning pain in the urethra; and difficult urination.

Disharmony in the Extraordinary Organs

Marrow and Brain   If marrow is deficient, the brain becomes unbalanced, and symptoms include ringing in the ears, vertigo, shakiness, poor eyesight and difficulty thinking. Weak bones and retarded bone growth also can occur.

Uterus   If Heart Xue is Deficient, the Heart Qi does not descend to the uterus, and periods may become irregular or stop altogether. Failure of Kidney Jing to descend to the uterus can result in infertility, irregular periods or complete cessation of menstruation.

Because of the dependence of the uterus on the Organ Systems, treatment for all menstrual and reproductive problems is through the Liver, Kidney, Spleen or Heart System and related primary and extraordinary channels.

THE EFFECT OF DISHARMONY ON THE CHANNELS

Channels are affected by disharmonies that are distinct from those afflicting Organ Systems and the Essential Substances. If you visit a practitioner who is solely an acupuncturist, then all treatment will be determined through the diagnosis of channel disharmonies.

When a pathogen causes disharmony in a channel, the acu-points become tender to the touch. The tender spots are useful in diagnosis, since they clue the practitioner to the location and nature of the imbalance along the channel and in the associated Organ System(s).

The following are the pathologies identified by Traditional Chinese Medicine that correspond to the twelve primary and eight extraordinary channels and the fifteen collaterals. Not all schools of acupuncture accept these indications for diagnosis and treatment.

PATHOLOGIES OF THE TWELVE PRIMARY CHANNELS

Each of the twelve primary channels is associated with distinct disharmonies. These disharmonies, which arise when the flow of Qi is disrupted, create symptoms in the part of the body through which the channel flows. Each channel has exterior and interior pathways. The exterior pathways are relatively near the surface of the skin and contain the acu-points; the interior pathways are relatively deep and cannot be needled directly.

Lung Channel of Hand-Taiyin

Symptoms associated with disharmonies of the Lung channel of hand-Taiyin (*tie-yin*) include cough, asthmatic breathing, coughing up blood, congested and sore throat, the feeling that a baby elephant is standing on your chest, pain in the neck, pain in the upper chest, and pain running along the lower section of the inside of the arm.

The Large Intestine Channel of Hand-Yangming

Symptoms associated with disharmonies of the Large Intestine channel of hand-Yangming (*yang-ming*) include nosebleeds, runny nose, toothaches, congested and sore throat, neck pain, pain in the front of the shoulder and the front edge of arm, noisy bowels, abdominal pain, diarrhea and dysentery.

After a decade of performing surgery, Sonia had developed chronic pain in her right wrist. It was diagnosed by an orthopedist as repetitive use syndrome and she was told her options were to have surgery or suffer progressive nerve damage. "I'm a Western doctor, through and through, but I figured I had nothing to lose by trying acupuncture. I never thought it would really work, but I was desperate."

She came to the clinic from out of town, saying she could only stick around for one treatment. She was diagnosed with an injury to the Large Intestine channel due to trauma. I suggested that she get a wrist splint, make changes in her surgical schedule, and I gave her an herbal trauma salve to apply to the wrist daily. She then had a thirty-minute acupuncture treatment with electrostimulation and moxibustion on her wrist.

A week later, she called the clinic to report that she was 80 to 90 percent better after the treatment. Six weeks later, when she was in town again, she received another treatment. She now reports a 95 percent improvement and has vowed that every time she comes to San Francisco, she'll get a tune-up treatment. She has also learned how to use self-care to avoid reinjury.

The Stomach Channel of Foot-Yangming

Symptoms associated with disharmonies of the Stomach channel of foot-Yangming (*yang-ming*) include noisy bowels, distended abdomen, edema, vomiting and stomach pain, hunger, bloody nose, a droopy mouth, congested and sore throat, chest and abdominal pain, pain along the outside of the leg, fever and mania.

The Spleen Channel of Foot-Taiyin

Symptoms associated with disharmonies of the Spleen channel of foot-Taiyin (*tie-yin*) include belching, vomiting, stomach pain, distended abdomen, loose stools, jaundice, an overall feeling of lethargy and heaviness, inflexibility and pain where the tongue attaches to the mouth, and swelling and cold along the inside of the knee and thigh.

The Heart Channel of Hand-Shaoyin

Symptoms associated with disharmonies of the Heart channel of hand-Shaoyin (*shouw-yin*) include heart pain, palpitations, pain in the chest and ribs, insomnia, night sweats, dry throat and thirst, hot palms and pain along the inside of the upper arm.

Small Intestine Channel of Hand-Taiyang

Symptoms associated with disharmonies of the Small Intestine channel of hand-Taiyang (*tie-yang*) include deafness, yellowing of the whites of the eyes, sore throat, swollen cheeks and throat, pain along the back edge of the shoulder and arm and lower abdomen distention and pain.

Bladder Channel of Foot-Taiyang

Symptoms associated with disharmonies of the Bladder channel of foot-Taiyang (*tie-yang*) include bed-wetting or trouble urinating, depression and mania, blocked and stuffy nose, teary eyes (particularly in the wind), runny nose, eye pain, bloody nose, headache, and pain along the bladder channel from the nape of the neck to the middle of the back of the legs.

The Kidney Channel of Foot-Shaoyin

Symptoms associated with disharmonies of the Kidney channel of foot-Shaoyin (*shouw-yin*) include bed-wetting, too-frequent urination, nocturnal emission, impotence, asthmatic breathing and coughing up blood, dry tongue, congested and sore throat, edema, lower back pain, irregular periods, pain along the back edge of the inside of the thigh, weak legs and hot soles of the feet.

Pericardium Channel of Hand-Jueyin

Symptoms associated with disharmonies of the Pericardium channel of hand-Jueyin (*joo-yin*) include heart pain, palpitations, tight chest and trouble breathing, emotional restlessness, depression and mania, flushed face, swelling in the armpits, arm spasms and hot palms.

The Triple Burner (Sanjiao) of Hand-Shaoyang

Symptoms associated with disharmonies of the Triple Burner (Sanjiao) of hand-Shaoyang (*shouw-yang*) include distended abdomen, bed-wetting, painful urination, deafness, ringing in the ears, pain at the outer edge of the eye, swollen cheeks, congested and sore throat, pain behind the ear, shoulder pain and pain in the back of the arm and elbow.

The Gallbladder Channel of Foot-Shaoyang

Symptoms associated with disharmonies of the Gallbladder channel of foot-Shaoyang (*shouw-yang*) include headache, pain at the outer edge of the eye, jaw pain, blurry vision, a bitter taste in the mouth, swelling and pain in the upper chest and armpit, pain along the outside of the chest and rib area and pain in the outside of the thigh and lower leg.

The Liver Channel of Foot-Jueyin

Symptoms associated with disharmonies of the Liver channel of foot-Jueyin (*joo-yin*) include low back pain, fullness in the chest, pain in the lower stomach, hernia, pain on the top of the head, dry throat, hiccups, bed-wetting, painful urination and mental disharmony.

PATHOLOGIES OF THE EIGHT EXTRAORDINARY CHANNELS

These channels are closely related to the Liver System, Kidney System, uterus, brain and marrow, and they serve to connect the twelve primary channels and regulate their Qi and Xue. The pathological manifestations listed here are based on the physiological functions and the area of each channel's influence. Work with them during self-massage and acupressure. They have a big role in disharmonies of women's reproductive cycle (see page 233).

Du Mai

Symptoms associated with disharmonies of the Du Mai (*do-my*) or Governing channel include stiff, painful spine; severe muscle spasm causing arching of the back; headache; and epilepsy.

Ren Mai

Symptoms associated with disharmonies of the Ren Mai (*ren-my*), the Conception channel, include vaginal discharge, irregular periods, infertility in women and men, hernia, nocturnal emission, bed-wetting, urinary retention, stomach, lower abdominal and genital pain.

Chong Mai

Symptoms associated with disharmonies of the Chong Mai (*chong-my*), the Penetrating channel, include spasm and pain in the abdomen, irregular periods, asthmatic breathing, infertility in women and men, and in my observations, emotional and physical problems arising from various forms of abuse.

Dai Mai

Symptoms associated with disharmonies of the Dai Mai (*die-my*), the Belt channel, include weak lower back, vaginal discharge, uterine prolapse, trouble moving hips and legs, weakness and muscular atrophy of lower limbs, and an unaccountable feeling like one is sitting in water.

Yangqiao Mai

Symptoms associated with disharmonies of the Yangqiao Mai (*yang-chow-my*), the Yang heel channel, include insomnia, redness and pain at the inside corner of the eye, pain in the back and lower back, turning out of the foot, spasm of the lower limbs and epilepsy.

Yinqiao Mai

Symptoms associated with disharmonies of the Yinqiao Mai (*yin-chow-my*), the Yin heel channel, include epilepsy, lethargy, pain in the lower abdomen, lower back and hip pain that causes referred pain in the pubic region, and leg spasms and inversion of the foot.

Yangwei Mai

Symptoms associated with disharmonies of the Yangwei Mai (*yang-way*), the Yang linking channel, include external symptoms such as chills and fever.

Yinwei Mai

Symptoms associated with disharmonies of the Yinwei Mai (*yin-way-my*), the Yin linking channel, include internal pain in chest and heart pain and stomachaches.

PATHOLOGIES OF THE 15 COLLATERALS

The collaterals branch off the primary channels with which they are associated. They strengthen the relationships between the paired internal and external channels and move Qi and Xue to organs and tissues in the body. When disharmony occurs, the collaterals compound the symptoms of the primary channel with which they are associated.

Collateral of the Lung Channel of Hand-Taiyin

Symptoms associated with disharmonies of this channel include hot palms and wrists, shortness of breath, bed-wetting and frequent urination.

Collateral of the Large Intestine Channel of Hand-Yangming

Symptoms associated with disharmonies of this channel include toothache, deafness, cold teeth and a stifling feeling in the chest and diaphragm.

Collateral of the Stomach Channel of Foot-Yangming

Symptoms associated with disharmonies of this channel include depression and mania, atrophy of muscles and weakness in lower leg, congested and sore throat, and sudden attack of hoarseness.

Collateral of the Spleen Channel of Foot-Taiyin

Symptoms associated with disharmonies of this channel include spasm of the abdomen, vomiting and diarrhea.

Collateral of the Heart Channel of Hand-Shaoyin

Symptoms associated with disharmonies of this channel include chest and diaphragm fullness and aphasia.

Collateral of the Small Intestine Channel of Hand-Taiyang

Symptoms associated with disharmonies of this channel include weak joints, muscular atrophy and impaired movement in the elbow and skin warts.

Collateral of the Bladder Channel of Foot-Taiyang

Symptoms associated with disharmonies of this channel include stuffed-up, runny nose, headache, back pain and bloody nose.

Collateral of the Kidney Channel of Foot-Shaoyin

Symptoms associated with disharmonies of this channel include low back pain, urinary retention, mental restlessness and a stifling sensation in the chest.

Collateral of the Pericardium Channel of Hand-Jueyin

Symptoms associated with disharmonies of this channel include heart pain and mental restlessness.

Collateral of the Triple Burner (Sanjiao) of Hand-Shaoyang

Symptoms associated with disharmonies of this channel include flaccidity or spasm on the inside of the elbow.

Collateral of the Gallbladder Channel of Foot-Shaoyang

Symptoms associated with disharmonies of this channel include cold feet, paralysis of legs and inability to stand upright.

Collateral of the Liver Channel of Foot-Jueyin

Symptoms associated with disharmonies of this channel include constant erection, itching in the pubic area, swollen testes and hernia.

Collateral of the Ren Mai

Symptoms associated with disharmonies of this channel include abdominal pain that exerts an outward pressure and itching of abdominal skin.

Collateral of the Du Mai

Symptoms associated with disharmonies of this channel include stiff spine, heavy sensation in the head and head tremor.

The Great Collateral of the Spleen

Symptoms associated with disharmonies of this channel include overall achiness, muscle pain and weakness in arm and leg joints.

PART TWO

THE HEALING PROCESS

CHAPTER FIVE

When You Visit a Chinese Medicine Practitioner

Evaluation and Diagnosis

When you go to a Chinese medicine practitioner, whether for treatment of an illness, acute pain, or to begin a program of preventive care, the doctor will follow a system of evaluation and diagnosis that depends on observation and questioning. In accordance with the philosophy of the Tao, diagnosis is a process of perceiving signs and symptoms and relating them to one another to reveal how they form patterns of harmony or disharmony. Each symptom or sign has meaning only in relationship to other signs and symptoms and to the whole of your mind/body/ spirit.

THE FOUR EXAMINATIONS

In order to begin to develop an accurate picture of your whole being, the Chinese medicine practitioner examines you, using the traditional Chinese method, called the Four Examinations: inquiring, looking, listening/smelling (these two seemingly different acts are grouped together—in Chinese they are the same word) and touching. This process of examination reveals which of the Eight Fundamental Patterns of disharmony are at work and what type of disharmony of the Essential Substances, Organ Systems and channels you may have.

The Four Examinations are sometimes done formally, but often the practitioner uses intuition and casual observation to create a vivid profile of a patient. Every gesture, word and attribute provides clues to a person's health and well-being.

Let's look at each step in the diagnostic process in more detail, breaking down the Four Examinations into their components, so you'll know what to expect.

INQUIRING

Step One: Asking Questions

The Chinese medicine doctor takes a great deal of time to ask you about yourself. Your answers allow the practitioner to benefit from the knowledge that you have, for no one can know your body as well as you do. Questioning allows the practitioner to observe your emotions, voice and self-presentation. Basic questions focus on:

- Your reaction to heat and cold
- Your patterns of perspiration
- If and when you experience headaches or dizziness
- What type of pain, if any, you may have
- Your bowel and bladder function
- Your thirst, appetite, and tastes
- Sleep patterns
- Your sexual functioning, sexual activity, and reproductive history
- General medical history
- General physical activity
- Emotions

LOOKING

Step Two: Evaluation of the Tongue

The tongue is the mirror of the body. Harmony and disharmony are reflected in the tongue's color, moisture, size, coating and the location of abnormalities.

Healthy Organ Systems and a lack of External Pernicious Influences produce a healthy tongue, which is pinkish red, neither dry nor too wet, fits perfectly within the mouth, moves freely and has a thin white coating.

Imbalances in the Organ Systems and/or invasion by Pernicious Influences produce an unhealthy tongue. External Pernicious Influences produce changes in the tongue coating. Interior problems, such as Organ System or Essential Substance disharmonies, produce changes in the tongue body.

When examining the tongue, the Chinese medicine doctor looks at the color of the tongue body, its size and shape, the color and thickness of its coating or fur, locations of abnormalities, and moistness or dryness of the tongue body and fur. These signs reveal not only overall states of health but correlate to specific organ functions and disharmonies, especially in the digestive system. To evaluate the tongue accurately, always do the examination in natural light.

Tongue Body   The tongue body is a fleshy mass and has color, texture, and shape independent from the apparent qualities of the tongue coating. A pale tongue body indicates Deficient Xue, Qi, or Yang or Excess Cold. An overly red tongue body indicates Excess Heat. A purple tongue indicates that Qi and/or Xue are not moving harmoniously and are stagnant. Pale purple means the Stagnation is related to Cold. Reddish purple is related to Stagnation of Heat. When the tongue is black or gray, it indicates extreme Stagnation; if black and dry, that indicates extreme Heat Stagnation; if black and wet, that indicates extreme Cold Stagnation. Bright red indicates Deficient Yin or Excess Heat. Dark red indicates Excess Heat. Cracks in a red tongue indicate Deficient Yin or Heat Injuring the Fluids. If the tongue is pale and cracked, there is Deficient Qi or Xue. Thorny eruptions of the buds on the tongue alert the doctor to Heat or Stagnant Xue.

Tongue Fur   The tongue's coating is best described as moss or fur. It arises when the Spleen causes tiny amounts of impure substances to drift upward to the tongue. When the Spleen and stomach are in balance, there is a uniform density of fur, with a slightly thicker area in the center of the tongue. Thick fur indicates excess. Thin fur is related to deficiency during illness, but is normal if you are well. Fur that is wet indicates Excess Jin-Ye (fluids) and/or a Deficient Yang. Dry fur is a sign of Excess Yang or Deficient Jin-Ye. A greasy fur is a sign of mucus or dampness in the body. If the fur looks peeled off or missing, it reveals Deficient Spleen or Yin or fluids. White, moist fur indicates Cold. Yellow fur means Heat. However, white fur, resembling cottage cheese, points to heat in the Stomach. Gray/black fur with a red body is associated with extreme Heat; gray/black fur with a pale body is a sign of extreme Cold.

Size and Shape   The healthy tongue rests comfortably in the mouth. It is neither too small nor too large. If a tongue is enlarged and flabby, it indicates Deficient Qi. If, in addition to being enlarged and flabby, the tongue has scalloped (or tooth-marked) edges, then it indicates dampness due to Deficient Qi or stagnation of fluids. If the tongue is enlarged and hard, it is a sign of Excess. If it swells so that it fills the mouth and is deep red, that means Excess Heat in Heart and Spleen are a problem. A small, thin tongue can indicate Deficient Yin or Xue.

Movement   A trembling, pale tongue indicates Deficient Qi. A flaccid tongue that is pale often reveals extreme Qi or Xue Deficiency. A flaccid tongue that is deep red reveals severe Yin Deficiency. A trembling, red tongue indicates interior Wind. If the tongue sits off-center in the mouth, early or full-blown Wind stroke may be present. A rigid tongue accompanies an Exterior Pernicious Influence and fever. This may indicate the invasion of the Pericardium by Heat and Mucus Obstructing the Heart Qi.

Location of Abnormalities   The location of disturbances on the tongue are vivid indications of where disharmonies in the mind/body/spirit are located. Certain organs are associated with the Upper, Middle and Lower Triple Burner, which are in turn associated with the front, middle and back sections of the tongue. For example, if there are red spots on the front third of the tongue, which is associated with the Upper Burner, this indicates that there is Heat in the Lungs. If the tip of the tongue is red, that indicates Heat in the Heart. Menstrual cramps, when as-

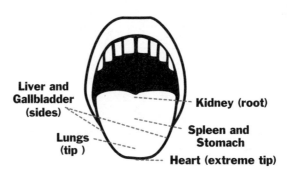

**Liver and
Gallbladder
(sides)**

Kidney (root)

**Lungs
(tip)**

**Spleen and
Stomach**

Heart (extreme tip)

**Areas of the Tongue and
Corresponding Organs**

sociated with Stagnant Xue, are often accompanied by purple spots on the edges of the tongue in the Liver/Gallbladder area.

The Role of Tongue Diagnosis   Not all tongue irregularities are indications of disharmony, however. Food and drugs may change the coating or color of the body of the tongue. For example, coffee yellows the coating and Pepto-Bismol turns the tongue black.

Furthermore, some people have minor, unchanging cracks on their tongue, which are considered normal. Others are born with what is called a geographic tongue, which is covered with severe cracks and covered with hills and valleys. This is considered normal by some practitioners, but a sign of congenital disharmony by others.

The way a tongue appears is not an absolute indicator of the location of the disharmony, but when taken as part of an overall pattern that includes a complete evaluation, it offers strong clues to the location of disharmony.

Step Three: Evaluation of Body Language—Styles of Movement, Posture and Self-Presentation

Seeking clues to possible Pernicious Influences, the practitioner looks for signs of heat or Cold influences, Excess or Deficiency, Yin or Yang disharmonies. If a person has a heavy-footed walk, loud voice and sits in a sloppy, spread-out posture, that may indicate Excess. If a person acts frail and weak, sits with shoulders slumped and is shy and receding, that may indicate a Deficiency. On the other hand, fast, jerky, impulsive movement and an outgoing personality indicate Heat. If combined with a full, red face, high energy and a loud voice, then both Heat and Excess may be at work. Cold, as you might suspect, is associated with slow but not sloppy movements and a pale face. When coupled with a low voice, shortness of breath, or passivity, Cold and Deficiency may be at work.

Step Four: Evaluation of Facial Color

When you are feeling off-balance or have a specific disharmony, facial colors offer clues to the nature and the severity of the imbalance.

There are several different methods of facial diagnosis: Korean, Japanese, Worsley School, even macrobiotic. The following evaluation of facial colors is derived from a combination of Traditional Chinese Medicine and Five Phases principles.[1] I have found this system provides accurate analysis.

TIP

In order to obtain a clear idea of what the various facial colors look like, always use natural light when examining your face in a mirror.

The Significance of Facial Colors

• If facial color is bright and fresh, then the disease is called floating and is on a superficial level.

• If the color is moist, neither wet nor dry, the disease is not severe and will be easy to treat.

• If the color is shallow and scattered over a large area, the number of days of the disease will be short.

• If the color is dark and cloudy, then the disease is sinking into the inner organs.

• If the color is dark, cloudy and dry, the disease is severe and will be difficult to cure.

• If the color is deep and accumulated in one spot, the disease is a long-term one.

Reading Between the Lines   Five colors appear on the face: red, green, yellow, white and black. Depending on a person's constitution, a healthy face may have one color that is more predominant than others, but several may be visible. To determine what colors are present in your face, always examine it in natural light. Look for the overall color tone; study the skin to see what tones appear from under the surface; look at any visible veins. For contrast, hold your hand up alongside your face.

Red is the color associated with the Heart Organ System and Xue. If the face is a fresh red, the Xue is Hot. If the face is dark red, the Xue is Stagnant. If it is light red, the Xue is Deficient.

Green is the color associated with the Liver System and circulation of the Xue. If veins on the face appear greenish purple, the Xue is Hot. If the veins appear greenish black, the Xue is Stagnant. If the condition is severe, the veins on the face appear black.

Yellow is the color associated with the Spleen System. If the face appears light yellow, then the Spleen system is Damp and Hot. If the face appears deep yellow,

Heat has accumulated. If it is dark yellow, Heat is the result of Xue Stagnation. Withered yellow indicates a Heat Deficiency.

White is the color associated with the Lung System, which regulates Qi, the breathing in of oxygen, and the exhalation of carbon dioxide. If a person is not able to exhale completely—as in emphysema—his or her face will take on a grayish white color. If the person inhales inadequately, then the face will appear pale and lusterless.

Black is the color associated with the Kidney System. If the face is cold and black, the Kidney System is not filtering Xue properly. If the face color is black but bright and moist, the condition can be treated. If the face is not shining, the condition is not good. If the face is withered, the Kidney System Yin is dry. If the face is cloudy and dark, the Kidney System Yang is dying.

Occasionally, there are combinations of colors. This further refines the evaluation. For example, if the color is red and white, both the Heart and Lung channels are involved.

BODY SIGNS

Take a couple of minutes to evaluate your facial color and tongue body and fur. For both facial colors and tongue, do an evaluation with a friend so you can compare the differences in skin tone and tongue qualities.

On your face, do you see black, white, green, yellow, and/or red? Is the color bright, moist, floating, shallow, cloudy, dark, or dry? Is your tongue trembling and pale, flaccid, or red? Is it enlarged and flabby or scalloped? Or is it enlarged and hard or thin and small?

LISTENING AND SMELLING

Step Five: Evaluation of Voice

Listening to the sound of a person's speech, breathing and cough can help identify a disharmony that results from one or more pernicious influence and pattern of disharmony. For example, if the voice is too loud and strident, that indicates Excess, as does the sudden onset of a violent cough. A weak, low voice that doesn't project and a weak cough indicate Deficiency. Losing your voice or hoarseness can indicate either Deficiency or Excess. Wheezing arises from Dampness.

Step Six: Evaluation of Smell

According to TCM theory, there are two main odors that clue a doctor to the origin of disharmony. A strong stench from secretions or excretions indicates Excess and Heat. A weaker odor indicates Deficiency and Cold.

Five Phases practitioners (see chapter 2, page 32) generally rely on smell more than TCM practitioners do. Each smell is associated with a phase and can indicate disharmony with the associated organ or among organs that are related through the Five Phases cycle. The smells used in Five Phases diagnosis are: goatish, associated with wood; burning, associated with fire; fragrant, associated with earth; rank, associated with metal; and rotten, associated with water.

TOUCHING

Step Seven: Evaluation of Pulses

There are twenty-eight pulse qualities that are essential to Traditional Chinese Medicine's process of evaluation and diagnosis. Learning to read pulses requires years of study and practice and is not something that can be done at home on yourself. However, your Chinese medicine practitioner will talk to you about your pulse diagnosis, and you will want to have a passing familiarity with the terminology that's used. The most common descriptions are: floating, slippery, choppy, wiry, tight, slow, rapid, thin, big, empty and full. (For a more detailed explanation of pulse diagnosis, see *The Web That Has No Weaver*, by Ted Kaptchuk, or Chinese texts listed in the resource appendix.)

Pulses are evaluated on a superficial, middle and deep level. The normal pulse resides at the middle level and is usually about four or five beats for each complete inhalation and exhalation of breath.

Disharmonies of the pulses indicate: the condition of Qi, Xue and Fluids; Organ System imbalance(s); the location of the imbalance(s); and the nature (Heat or Cold) of the disease, along with many other qualities.

For example, a wiry pulse may indicate that the Liver System has Stagnant Qi. However, there are no absolute meanings to pulses. They contribute to a diagnosis only when viewed in context with other diagnostic techniques.

Step Eight: Evaluation of Sensitivity to Touch

Palpation of acupuncture points and channels can trigger, increase, or reduce pain and indicate disharmony in the associated channels and Organ Systems.

• If you have a pain you can't pinpoint, that indicates Stagnant Qi. Stagnant Qi is also indicated by a pain that moves around.

• If the pain is fixed, it may indicate Stagnant Xue.

• Pain that feels better with pressure is due to Deficiency.

• Pain that feels worse with pressure is due to Excess.

• Pain that feels better with warmth is associated with Cold.

Palpation of the body does not have to be confined to the twelve channels', fifteen collaterals' or eight extraordinary channels' acupuncture points. Ear acupuncture points are also powerful tools for diagnosis and provide refined clues to the sources of disharmony. They are also useful for self-massage (see pages 179 and 180). Reflexology, while not a traditional Chinese method of diagnosis and treatment, is another useful tool at this stage of diagnosis (see page 191).

THE NEXT STEP

Now that you have an understanding of the basics of Chinese medicine and what to expect if you go for acupuncture or herbal therapy, you may be ready to make an appointment to see a Chinese medicine practitioner. The following guidelines may help you find a qualified practitioner.

SELECTING A PRACTITIONER

When you are selecting an acupuncturist, herbalist, or a Chinese medicine doctor, the two most important factors to consider are the doctor's training and your goals.

Training

In order to gain the full benefit of Chinese medicine therapy, the practitioner who administers the treatment(s) should have reputable training and a keen sense of the philosophical underpinning of Chinese medicine.

The best way to determine if a practitioner meets those standards is to ask a lot of questions about his or her training, length of practice, scope of practice, specializations, attitudes about wellness and disharmony and understanding of Chinese medicine philosophy.

Meeting Basic Standards

The Taoist system of belief is not some fancy window dressing that can be cast aside. It is part and parcel of Chinese medicine treatments. No particular Chinese medicine therapy, such as acupuncture or herbal remedies, can deliver its full healing potential if it is separated from the philosophical context of the Tao.

In addition, you want to find a practitioner who is schooled in the Chinese medicine therapies that you want to use. There are practitioners who are licensed acupuncturists (L.Ac.) but who do not offer herbal therapy; there are others who are herbalists but provide no acupuncture; there are licensed acupuncturists who also have training as herbalists; and there are doctors of Oriental medicine who provide acupuncture and herbal therapy.

Every acupuncturist should be licensed (in states with licensing requirements) or certified. In more than half the states there are state licensing boards and nationally there is the National Commission for the Certification of Acupuncturists (NCCA). You may call the commission (see listing in the appendix) for a listing of certified acupuncturists in your area.

If you live in a state without a state licensing board, it is particularly important that your acupuncturists have a certificate from the NCCA. Acupuncture degrees in this country come from accredited schools of acupuncture and Traditional Chinese Medicine schools and colleges.

Your herbalist (who may also be your acupuncturist) should have either a certificate of training or a long-standing reputation and years of experience. Many schools train people in herbal medicine, but there is no independent licensing for Chinese herbalists. Since 1982, California is the only state that requires practitioners to take an exam in both acupuncture and herbal therapy to be licensed to practice acupuncture. The NCCA does offer an herbal certification, but it doesn't lead to licensure.

Your Goals

You also want to decide if you are looking for a primary care physician, someone to work with your primary care doctor, or simply someone who can provide short-term treatment for a specific complaint.

If you are looking for a primary care physician, I recommend someone who is knowledgeable about all aspects of Chinese medicine and Western medical procedures; someone who will know when to refer you for Western evaluations and testing, and someone who is willing to work with a Western doctor, if doing so provides you with the best therapy.

To sum up what to look for in a primary care Chinese medicine practitioner:

1. Someone who does not make promises to cure disorders and diseases for which there is no cure (applies to all practitioners, no matter what you use them for)
2. Someone who understands that there may be many different modalities that work for an individual and does not insist that his or her way is the only right or good way to go
3. Someone who has a bedside manner that pleases you (What pleases some people most is ability, and they don't care about personality at all. That's fine. For others, a more personal relationship is important. You should make that individual decision.)
4. Someone who is able to explain what she or he is doing from both a Chinese and a Western viewpoint—or is at least willing to find out about the alternative perspective when necessary
5. A practitioner who is not unconditionally opposed to any drug therapy in conjunction with acupuncture or herbal treatment, and who understands the interactions of drugs and herbs
6. Someone who will work with medical doctors and other practitioners

In cases of serious illnesses, you want to select a practitioner who understands Western medical terminology and concepts of the immune system, viruses and cancer, as well as Chinese concepts, if you are going for treatment of these problems.

If you have HIV, chronic hepatitis, or CFIDS (chronic fatigue immune deficiency syndrome), be sure that the practitioner's attitude is that you can live with this chronic, manageable viral infection and that acupuncture and herbs may help you be more successful in that process.

RECEIVING TREATMENT

When you select a practitioner and go for treatment, you don't surrender control of your health. Chinese medicine recognizes that we each possess the tools we need to preserve or reclaim good health. The good (or excellent) practitioner simply acts as the guide, helping to coax the body's own defenses to prevent or mend disharmony.

There are four basic healing techniques that the practitioner may suggest as treatments: acupuncture and moxibustion, herbal therapy, dietary therapy, and Qi Gong exercise/meditation. A brief description follows here, and each therapy is discussed in detail in the following chapters.

Dietary Therapy

Chinese dietary therapy uses foods to strengthen digestion, increase energy and balance the body's energy. Dietary therapy is often used prior to or in conjunction with other therapies to increase the effectiveness of these treatments.

Acupuncture and Moxibustion

Classic acupuncture is the art of inserting fine, sterile, metal filiform needles into certain points along the channels and collaterals (tributaries of the channels) in order to control the flow of the Qi. These days, practitioners also use electrostimulation of the needles, lasers and even ultrasound to stimulate the points.

Acupuncture is well-known for its effectiveness as a painkiller. Even more powerful is its ability to alter the flow of the Qi so that the body can heal itself when attacked by pathogens that trigger disharmony. Acupressure and massage are subsets of acupuncture.

Moxibustion, the burning of the herb moxa (Chinese mugwort) over channel points and certain areas of the body, is used to warm, tonify and stimulate. It also induces the smooth flow of the Essential Substances, prevents diseases and preserves health. Doing moxa regularly on specific acupuncture points is said to promote strength and longevity. In fact, an old Chinese saying is, "Never take a long journey with a person who does not have a Moxa scar on [the acupuncture point called] Stomach 36."

Chinese Herbal Medicine

Herbal medicine is actually a misnomer. Although the overwhelming majority of medicinal substances come from plants, some are derived from minerals and animals. Whatever their origin, they are used to balance the mind/body/spirit as well as to reverse disease processes. Most Chinese herbs should only be taken under the supervision of a trained herbalist.

Qi Gong Exercise/Meditation

Qi Gong, the Chinese art of exercise/meditation, uses dynamic movements and still postures in combination with mental and spiritual concentration to influence the flow of Qi. It is a powerful preventive therapy and can help remedy disharmony in the Organ Systems and the channels.

CHAPTER SIX

You Are What You Eat

The Four Principles of Chinese Medicine Dietary Practices

Wholeness = **Dietary Guidelines** + Herbs + Acupuncture + Qi Gong

Diet, acupuncture, herbs and exercise/meditation are the four therapeutic tools of Chinese medicine: They are used to build, maintain and restore wholeness in mind/body/spirit.

Diet is extremely important because every day what you eat either nourishes or dilutes your Essential Substances.

Grain (Gu) Qi enters your body through food. Combined with Respiratory (Kong) Qi, which enters the body through breathing, and Prenatal (Yuan) Qi, which is inherited from parents, it forms Normal (Zheng) Qi, the wellspring and companion of all movement in the body. Normal Qi assists the release of stored Nutritive (Ying) Qi from food. This process underlies the far-reaching power of diet therapy.

What you eat shapes your Shen. Shen, the spirit, is the driving force that makes us uniquely human. It enters the body from the parents before birth. After birth, Shen is dependent on Qi and on what you eat to retain its vitality.

Your diet has an impact on your Jing. Jing is the basis of life—Qi emerges from Jing, but Qi also transforms food into postnatal Jing so that life can be nurtured and continue to blossom. Since a balanced diet builds healthy Qi, Jing is affected by what you eat.

A balanced diet maintains the unique relationship between Qi and Xue. It allows Qi to influence Xue and Xue to nurture Qi.

DIETARY PRINCIPLE NUMBER ONE: YOU ARE WHAT YOU EAT... AND WHAT YOU DON'T EAT

Food has tremendous powers in Chinese medicine—powers that extend far beyond the Western concept of food as fuel, providing calories, carbohydrates, protein, fat, vitamins and minerals. These powers are defined as energetics, which **cool or warm** the metabolism and Organ Systems, **moisturize or dry** the Organ Systems, and **increase or decrease** the flow of Qi, Jing, and Xue.

A healthy diet harnesses these energetics by combining foods that balance each other so that no one energetic influence becomes too strong.

If your diet contains an **imbalance** of energetics, your various Organ Systems and your Qi, Jing, Shen and Xue are subjected to more of a drying than a moisturizing influence or more of a cooling than a warming influence. This can cause stagnation or depletion of your Qi, Jing, and Xue and disharmony of Shen. You then become vulnerable to diseases and to emotional and spiritual discontent.

To balance energetics, eat warm foods to keep the digestive process working well. Don't eat too many raw foods. Despite common beliefs, they are not closer to nature and do not contain better nutrition. Chinese medicine sees raw foods as depleting. They may cause a Cold Damp condition since your body has to spend extra energy and heat to "cook" the food in your stomach. In my practice, I see the wreckage caused by overconsumption of raw foods: people with no energy and a constant chill who can't figure out why they don't feel good. It may take aggressive dietary therapy to rebalance the body after a diet of too many raw foods. The only people who should eat raw foods in higher than the recommended amounts are those who are very hot.

Chew each bite of food carefully to make the digestive process easier and to conserve the digestive fire. This fire is produced by the Central Qi, which warms the central Organ Systems so they have the power to digest food. Cold food cools that inner warmth and that's why it's not good to eat too many cold or raw foods.

Don't stuff yourself. Overeating overwhelms the digestive fire and causes Stagnation and disease.

Drink scant liquid during meals or you'll drown the digestive fires.

Avoid iced and frozen foods.

Eat organic, unprocessed foods as much as possible. The elimination of pesticides, hormones, antibiotics and other chemical residues in vegetables, meats, and dairy increases available Qi, removes antagonists to your overall health and makes food taste better. Obviously, this is not a component of Traditional Chinese Medicine; in ancient times, all food was organic. But today, with the proliferation of harmful chemical additives to food, we must add it to the top of our list of most important dietary considerations.

FOOD FLAVORS AND ENERGETICS

Warm Foods

Anchovy—sweet
Basil—spicy
Bay leaf—spicy
Black pepper—spicy
Brown sugar—sweet
Butter—sweet
Capers—spicy
Cherry—sweet
Chestnut—sweet
Chicken—sweet
Chicken livers—sweet
Coconut milk—sweet
Coriander—spicy
Dill seed—spicy
Fennel seed—spicy
Garlic—spicy
Ginger, fresh—spicy
Leek—spicy
Litchi—sweet & sour
Mussels—salty
Mustard greens—spicy
Mutton—sweet
Nutmeg—spicy
Onion—spicy
Peach—sweet & sour
Pine nuts—sweet
Rosemary—spicy
Safflower—spicy
Scallion—spicy & bitter
Shrimp—sweet
Sorghum—sweet
Spearmint—spicy & sweet
Squash—sweet
Strawberry—sweet & sour
Sweet potato—sweet
Sweet rice—sweet
Vinegar—sour & bitter
Walnut—sweet

Hot Foods

Cayenne—spicy
Ginger, dried—spicy
Soybean oil—spicy & sweet
Trout—sour

Cool Foods

Apple—sweet
Banana—sweet
Barley—sweet & salty
Buckwheat—sweet
Celery—sweet & bitter
Cucumber—sweet
Eggplant—sweet
Gluten—sweet
Lettuce—sweet & bitter
Millet—sweet & salty
Mushroom—sweet
Pear—sweet
Peppermint—spicy
Radish—spicy & sweet
Sesame oil—sweet
Soybean—sweet
Spinach—sweet
Swiss chard—sweet
Tangerine—sweet & sour
Tofu—sweet
Watercress—spicy & sweet
Wheat—sweet
Wheat bran—sweet

Cold Foods

Agar—sweet
Asparagus—sweet & bitter
Clams—salty
Crab—salty
Kelp—salty
Mango—sweet & sour
Mulberry—sweet
Mung bean sprouts—sweet
Nori—sweet & salty
Octopus—sweet & salty
Persimmon—sweet
Plantain—sweet
Romaine lettuce—bitter
Salt—salty
Seaweed—salty
Tomato—sweet & sour
Watermelon—sweet

Neutral Foods

Adzuki beans—sweet & sour
Alfalfa—bitter
Almond—sweet
Beef—sweet
Beet—sweet
Cabbage—sweet
Carrot—sweet
Cheese—sweet & sour
Eggs (chicken)—sweet
Coconut meat—sweet
Corn—sweet
Duck—sweet
Figs—sweet
Grapes—sweet & sour
Honey—sweet
Kidney beans—sweet
Milk—sweet
Olives—sweet & sour
Oysters—sweet & salty
Papaya—sweet & bitter
Peanuts—sweet
Peanut oil—sweet
Peas—sweet
Pineapple—sweet
Plum—sweet & sour
Pork—sweet & salty
Potato—sweet
Pumpkin—sweet
Raspberry—sweet
Rice—sweet
Rice bran—spicy & sweet
Rye—bitter
Sardines—sweet & salty
Shark—sweet & salty
String beans—sweet
Sugar (refined)—sweet
Turnips—spicy & sweet
Whitefish—sweet
Yam—sweet

FOOD FLAVORS AND ENERGETICS *(cont.)*

Sweet

Adzuki beans—& sour
Almond
Anchovy
Beef
Beet
Brown sugar
Butter
Cabbage
Carrot
Cheese—& sour
Cherry
Chestnut
Chicken
Chicken livers
Coconut
Meat
Coconut milk
Corn
Cucumber
Duck
Eggplant
Eggs (chicken)
Figs
Gluten
Grapes—& sour
Honey
Kidney beans
Lettuce—& bitter
Litchi—& sour
Mango—& sour
Milk
Millet—& salty
Mulberry
Mung bean sprouts
Mushroom

Mutton
Nori—& salty
Octopus—& salty
Olives—& sour
Oysters—& salty
Papaya—& bitter
Peach—& sour
Peanut oil
Peanuts
Pear
Persimmon
Pineapple
Pine nuts
Plantain
Plum—& sour
Pork—& salty
Potato
Pumpkin
Raspberry
Rice
Sardines—& salty
Sesame oil
Shark—& salty
Shrimp
Sorghum
Soybean
Spinach
Squash
Strawberry—& sour
String beans
Sugar (refined)
Sweet rice
Sweet potato
Swiss chard
Tangerine—& sour
Tofu

Tomato—& sour
Turnip—& spicy
Walnut
Watermelon
Wheat
Wheat bran
Whitefish
Yam

Spicy

Basil
Bay leaf
Black pepper
Capers
Cayenne
Coriander
Dill seed
Fennel seed
Garlic
Ginger, dried
Ginger, fresh
Leek
Mustard greens
Nutmeg
Onion
Peppermint
Radish—& sweet
Rice bran—& sweet
Rosemary
Safflower
Scallion—& bitter
Soybean oil—& sweet
Spearmint—& sweet
Watercress—& sweet

Sour

Trout
Vinegar—& bitter

Salty

Clams
Crab
Kelp
Mussels
Salt
Seaweed

Bitter

Alfalfa
Romaine
Rye
Shrimp

FOOD FLAVORS

Chinese medicine dietary practice also discusses the impact of food in terms of five flavors: sour, bitter, sweet, spicy, and salty. Each flavor has a hot and cold quality. There is a warm sour and a cool sour, a hot bitter and a cold bitter, and so on. A balanced diet is generally composed of mostly sweet, warm foods; cold, spicy, bitter, salty and sour are best eaten as accents. As a general rule: a little of any flavor tonifies; a salty flavor concentrates; sour contracts; bitter descends; sweet expands; and spicy disperses. There are no flavors that are bad except in excess or when you are fighting a disharmony.

> If people pay attention to the five flavors and blend them well, Qi and Xue will circulate freely and breath and bones will be filled with the essence of life.
>
> From the *Nei Jing*

You can use your own reactions to flavor as an indicator of what is out of balance in your body. For example, if you have an unusual craving for sweets, your earth is out of harmony. If you have an aversion to sour, your wood is affected. Eating too much salty food could negatively impact water, and an excess of bitter or pungent foods can cause disruption of the metal and fire channels and Organ Systems.

DIETARY PRINCIPLE NUMBER TWO: MOST OF YOUR FOOD SHOULD BE EATEN IN SEASON

DIET AND THE RHYTHMS OF THE EXTERNAL WORLD

Food gains power to maintain health from its relationship to the external world. Food, the fuel of the mind/body/spirit, should be taken into the body in a pattern that's attuned to the rhythms of the environment. This perspective is based on the Tao, the Chinese philosophy of the unity and interrelationship between the external and internal worlds.

As you look around the outside world, you can see that in the spring, energy moves up. In the summer, it moves out. In the autumn, energy moves down; in the winter, it moves inward. Likewise, green, sprouting vegetables move energy up. Spices, flowers and leaves have outward moving energy. Root vegetables have downward moving energy. Grains, seeds and nuts have inward moving energy.

To reap the benefits of food's energetic relationship to the seasons, you may want to eat foods in their own season when their power is strongest or in the season before to prepare your body for the coming season.

DIETARY PRINCIPLE NUMBER THREE: MODERATION AND VARIETY IN DIET ARE ESSENTIAL FOR A BALANCED MIND/BODY/SPIRIT

CREATING A BALANCED DIET

A balanced diet results from a combination of the foods you eat and the way you prepare, eat and think about your food. You could not create the perfect diet pill that combined all the energetics needed to achieve wholeness and harmony. Food energetics are not simply the result of chemistry, they are also a result of spiritual forces. The power of food—positive and negative—to influence your mind/body/ spirit is affected by how it is prepared, served and eaten.

THE SPIRIT OF A BALANCED DIET

There is not a list of good foods and bad foods. Too much of a healthy food is unhealthy. You can overdo it on broccoli or brown rice. Sugars aren't unhealthy. Too much or very refined sugar is. Meat (organic) isn't unhealthy. Too much meat is.

Balance comes from eating a variety of foods, including grains, vegetables, meats, fruits and dairy, each in moderation. If you do that, you can pretty much eat what you want.

The modern American diet-crazy notion that you should only eat from a roster of mildly unappealing, healthy foods and avoid bad foods is ill-advised. If you have one bite of chocolate, you haven't sinned. You can have your cake and eat it, too— in moderation. If your diet is balanced, your habits flexible, and your inclinations moderate, you have little to worry about.

As important as moderation is in achieving balance, it is also important to strive for the proper attitude toward food. Food prepared as a gift, served calmly, eaten with respect and digested in a harmonious atmosphere bestows positive benefits. Food slapped together without regard or with resentment, served as quickly as possible, gobbled down, or eaten while driving, watching TV, or even reading cannot be assimilated healthfully. If you eat fast food or if you eat food fast, you're better off fasting than feasting.

To achieve the spirit of a balanced diet:

1. Eat in a peaceful setting.
2. Relax before you begin to eat. Take a deep breath. Appreciate the food: its existence, its aroma, its appearance.
3. Eat slowly enough to chew adequately.
4. Eat with others whose company you enjoy.
5. Eat at regular times.

BODY SIGNS

The first step to improving harmony and balance through diet is to become aware of your current eating patterns. Think about which of these foods you eat most often.

Red Meat: How many times a week? _____

Chicken: How many times a week? _____

Fish: How many times a week? _____

Vegetables: How many times a day? _____

Beans: How many times a week? _____

Grains: How many times a day? _____

Dairy: How many times a day? _____

STAYING FLEXIBLE

It's so easy to get fanatic about diet. But rigidity about how you eat is itself a disease-producing behavior, even if you're being rigid about eating healthy foods. Health depends on a graceful adaptability to your surroundings and the ability to nourish yourself, even if the perfect foods aren't available.

In our food-obsessed, food-unhealthy culture, it's easy to misinterpret the Chinese medicine perspective on diet. For example, people sometimes use the five flavors in combination with the Five Phases and create artificial rules such as: Sour is associated with wood and spring is associated with wood, so you should eat sour things in the spring.

Chinese medicine doesn't work that way; that's too pat. Dietary therapy is a guide to help you find balance and moderation. It does not establish rigid do's and don'ts, rights and wrongs.

THE APPLICATION OF A BALANCED MEAL PLAN

How many times a day you eat is highly individual. Some people do better grazing on small meals throughout the day, especially if they have trouble maintaining their blood sugar levels. Others are happy with the traditional three meals a day. Some people find they run best with two meals a day. You want to follow what works for you, but as you begin to practice Chinese diet and receive acupuncture and herbal therapy from a Chinese medicine practitioner, you may find that your body becomes more balanced and needs fuel less frequently.

For those who follow the traditional three squares a day, here's a plan to help guide you.

Meal one: Eat a moderate amount of food—mostly grains—within two hours of waking up. Some sources also recommend protein in the morning. This meal should be made up of cooked, warming foods that stimulate your Qi.

Meal two: The largest meal of the day, this should combine grains with a small to moderate amount of high-grade protein such as soy and beans or a small amount of meat. A great variety of foods is the best. If indicated by your constitution or your practitioner's diagnosis, raw cool foods such as salads or fruits should be eaten now.

Meal three: The smallest meal of the day, this should not contain stimulating high-protein or spicy food. Chinese medicine also advises against eating within three hours of going to bed so that you can fully digest your food before retiring.

COMPOSITION OF MEALS

No matter how many times a day you eat or what adjustments you have to make to circumstances, you want to follow a basic balance of foods: 75 percent of your calories from grains, vegetables, and legumes (grains should account for two-thirds of this and vegetables and legumes for the other third); fruits should be about 10 percent of your daily calorie intake; and dairy and protein—including meats—should add up to about 10 percent.

PERCENTAGE OF FOODS IN BALANCED DIET PLAN

Grains: 50%	Vegetables: 20% Legumes: 5%	Fruits: 10%	Protein: 10%	Oil, sweets, and fat:<5%

BODY SIGNS

To help you take control of your dietary habits, try writing down everything you eat for a full day. Include all meals and snacks, sodas, juices, water and coffee. Compare that day's diet with the suggested diet in the chart above. Did you eat 50% of your calories in grains? A quarter of your calories in vegetables and legumes?

EATING MORE LEGUMES AND GRAINS

In Chinese medicine, one way that Qi enters the body is through Grain Qi, which indicates how important grains are to the health of the mind/body/spirit. Our modern diet has moved away from a focus on grains, but around the world, they are the basic food for most indigenous cuisines. They provide building blocks for protein and many of the essential vitamins and minerals.

You may want to expand your diet to include new types of grains such as couscous, millet, kasha, oats, rye, barley, wild rice, or brown rice. If you take the time to discover the many varieties that are available, you'll find it is much easier to make grains a central feature of your diet.

Grains are enhanced when combined with legumes such as limas, kidney beans, black beans, garbanzos, fava beans, white beans, pinto beans, navy beans, lentils, adzuki beans, soybeans, or split peas. In Western nutritional terms, the combination of grains and beans forms complete proteins.

Many people come into the clinic who don't know how to cook and are frustrated in their attempts to improve their diet because they eat out or get take-out food all the time. These basic recipes will help you prepare legumes or grains at home.

BARLEY
1 cup barley
3 cups water
1 tablespoon oil
1 pinch sea salt

Soak barley in cold water to cover, for 10–15 minutes. After soaking, pour off
    water and rinse with clear water twice.
Boil water and add oil and salt.
Add barley to boiling water. Cook for 1 minute.
Reduce to slow simmer and cook 1¼–1½ hours.
Stir occasionally during cooking.

Serves 3 or 4.
Good in soups, casseroles, or for breakfast.

MILLET (HULLED)
1 cup millet
1 cup water
1 pinch sea salt

Rinse millet 3 times under cold water.
Boil water and add sea salt. Add millet.
Boil millet for 1 minute.
Reduce to slow simmer and cook for at least 45 minutes.

Serves 2 or 3.
Good in casseroles, loafs, mixed with rice or vegetables.

COUSCOUS (CRACKED WHEAT)
1 cup couscous
2½ cups water
1 pinch sea salt

Rinse couscous 2 or 3 times.
Bring water to a boil. Add salt.
Add couscous to boiling water. Cover pot.
Reduce heat and slow simmer for 15 minutes.

Serves 2 or 3.
Good for casseroles, baking, desserts.

BEANS

Beans from a can are often high in fat, salt and sugar and low in vitamins. The following provides a simple guide to a wide variety of freshly cooked beans.

ADZUKI BEANS

Soak in enough water to cover, overnight. Boil in 3–4 cups water for 1½–2 hours.

Delicate flavor; combines well with rice, millet, squash, or onion.

BLACK BEANS

Soak overnight in enough water to cover. Boil in 3–4 cups water for 1½–2 hours.

Rich, earthy flavor; good with rice and in soups.

GARBANZOS (CHICKPEAS)

Soak in enough water to cover, overnight. Boil in 3–4 cups water 1–2 hours.

Nutty flavor; works well with curry; good in soups and salads.

KIDNEY BEANS

Soak overnight in enough water to cover. Boil in 3–4 cups water 1½–2 hours.

Bland; works well in soups, stews, salads.

LENTILS

No soaking. Boil in 2 cups water for 30–45 minutes.

Mild; good in soups, salads and with grains.

LIMA BEANS

Soak. Boil in 2 cups water for 45 minutes–1½ hours.

Good in soups and casseroles.

PINTO BEANS

Soak overnight. Cooking time: 1½–2 hours.

Mild, earthy flavor.

RED BEANS

Soak. Cooking time: 1½–2 hours.

Distinctive and savory; especially good with rice; good in soups, salads and stews.

SOYBEANS

Soak overnight. Cooking time: at least 3 hours.

Bland; best in casseroles, salads; highest in protein.

SPLIT PEAS

No soaking. Cooking time: 30–45 minutes.

Great in soups.

NAVY BEANS:

Soak. Cooking time: 1½–2 hours at a slow simmer.

Mild taste; best in soups or casseroles.

DIET AS PREVENTIVE MEDICINE

Chinese medicine's dietary practices form the basis for effective preventive medicine. When you eat foods that maintain the flow of Qi and the harmonious functioning of the Organ Systems, the immune system remains strong, bones and muscles remain flexible and supportive, digestion is good, the skin is healthy, the mind and spirit remain clear, and stress and anger dissipate.

However, as with so many Chinese medicine concepts, the effect of diet on bodily functions is not linear and cannot be viewed as a process of cause and effect: Instead, the association between food, Qi, Jing, Shen, Xue, the Organ Systems, and digestion depends on each element's influence over and reaction to the other elements.

This feedback mechanism is reflected in the role of the Spleen and Stomach Systems, which govern digestion and assimilation of food. The Stomach System releases the energy stored in food and the Spleen System distributes the food energy through the body. This maintains a harmonious flow of Qi, which in turn helps nourish the Spleen and Stomach Systems with an ample supply of Essential Substances, keeping them in balance. Without a well-balanced diet, the entire network of interdependence is interrupted.

You can also see the delicate yet powerful interdependence of diet and healthy (or unhealthy) Organ Systems when you look at the relationship between diet and the Triple Burner System, particularly the Middle Burner.

Food keeps the Middle Burner balanced so it maintains a strong Middle Burner fire. This warms the center and allows for proper digestion. If the fire becomes weak through lack of proper foods then the Middle Burner is forced to supplement its fire with energy drawn from the Lower Burner. When that happens, Kidney fire, which is fueled by the Lower Burner, may become depleted. That, in turn, can cause anxiety, imbalance, or agitation in the mind and spirit. Agitation in the mind and spirit can interfere with proper digestion. Before you know it, you've become trapped in a cycle of depletion and disharmony affecting body/mind/spirit—all because your diet was not balanced and couldn't support the Middle Burner's fire.

DIETARY PRINCIPLE NUMBER FOUR: FOOD IS POWERFUL MEDICINE

STAGES AND AGES OF DIETARY GUIDES

To reap the preventive benefits of Chinese medicine's dietary practices, you want to adjust your eating habits (and your family's) to the stages and ages of life. Infancy, adolescence, maturity and old age each have unique dietary requirements.

Infants and Young Children

Infants and children are immature energetically, although they do have Excess Qi and usually run a little warm. The Middle Burner is very sensitive, and the Triple Burner is not very strong. Because the Middle Burner Qi (Central Qi) is not strong, Spleen Qi weakness can develop, leading to Dampness. As a result, infants are likely to produce phlegm.

Before six months of age, feed only breast milk. From six to twelve months, breast milk is the most healthful food. If you use other milks, don't give any dairy before one year of age or soy before five or six months. Once you begin using soy, combine it with rice milk. Soy milk is too cooling for children and may produce a Damp condition (loose stools) that can aggravate allergies, cause runny nose, croup and diaper rashes. Use soy with rice milk or rice milk alone.

The first solid food to give a child—while still breast-feeding—is organic, whole-grain rice. Cook one cup of rice in five cups water to make a very watery gruel. Other foods can be added when breast-feeding stops.

Young children's diets should contain easy-to-digest, warming foods such as cooked vegetables, a modicum of well-cooked rice and only a little meat or meat broth. They need things that strengthen the Spleen, such as warming and neutral foods, which include carrots, string beans, yam, and potatoes. See the charts on pages 81–82 for other examples.

Young children should not be fed too much meat or grains since they may not completely digest them and that produces phlegm. Wheat, corn and dairy also create congestion and dampness.

Fruits, raw foods and cold drinks from the refrigerator are too cooling. Serve foods warm and beverages at room temperature.

Teens

Adolescents need lots of food to thrive. This is when the fire of sex, Kidney fire, is surging.

Adolescents should stay away from hot, spicy, or excessively sweet or oily foods, which force Heat to rise from the Stomach. This causes acne and emotional ups and downs, which are the plague of so many teenagers. Although for a healthy Spleen, everyone has to eat warming foods, teens do well to increase slightly the amount of cool or neutral foods they consume.

Adults

Mature individuals should eat a diverse diet with a full range of energetics to maintain their vigor. In people over forty, the Jing becomes depleted. In old age, the Kidney fire declines. Yin is consumed. As the Kidney fire becomes exhausted, the Middle Burner fire also becomes weak. The diet should return to the simple, easy-to-digest foods of the very young. Foods that are cool or cold are to be avoided, and moderation becomes ever more important to maintain energy.

Adults and especially the elderly should avoid eating more than two or three types of food at any one meal. That taxes the digestive fires. It is especially important not to overeat. Stagnation and disharmony follow, and it's harder and harder to restore balance. Food should be eaten in a relaxed atmosphere and never when you're upset.

These are the basics of healthful, well-balanced dietary practices. They provide protection against disease and help maintain vigor at all ages. But Chinese medicine's dietary guides can do far more than maintain health and prevent disease. They are also used to treat diseases and disorders. See Chapter 7, page 95, for details.

A CUP OF TEA

Tea is both a medicine and a beverage, an excuse for socializing and for solitary contemplation. Since the twelfth century B.C., it has occupied a special place in Chinese culture and was so valuable that it was used instead of money in business transactions well into this century.

As a folk medicine, tea has been used to help heal cuts and infections, soothe

the stomach, clarify the skin and energize the mind and spirit. An ancient Chinese proverb could be translated:

Drinking a daily cup of tea
Will surely starve the apothec'ry.[1]

The healing properties of tea have been confirmed by current research. Tea is known to contain polyphenols, which stimulate digestion. Research in China indicates polyphenols also may work as anticancer agents and enhance immune strength. Green tea, particularly lung ching, may be the most efficacious. In China and Japan, those who drink the most tea have the lowest incidence of stomach cancer. Tea also contains essential oils that may reduce circulating lipids and ease digestion, and it contains caffeine, which in small quantities can help circulate Xue and invigorate the mind. Although addiction to caffeine is not healthy, tea has less caffeine than coffee, and that can be reduced further by cutting the brewing time. Black tea that is steeped for five minutes contains twice the caffeine of tea that has steeped for three minutes.

COMPARATIVE CAFFEINE LEVELS

2 oz. espresso	60–69 mg caffeine
6 oz. drip coffee	60–180 mg caffeine
6 oz black tea, fermented	25–110 mg caffeine
6 oz. oolong, semifermented	12–55 mg caffeine
6 oz. green tea, unfermented	6–18 mg caffeine

Other health benefits indicated in recent research studies include green tea's cold-fighting and cavity-preventing abilities (it contains fluoride and has high levels of vitamin C). Pu-erh is a form of black tea renowned for its medicinal properties, particularly in easing indigestion and diarrhea. Modern studies indicate that it also reduces cholesterol and/or triglycerides.

Types of Tea

There are three types of Chinese tea, which are differentiated by how fermented they are. The word *fermented,* however, is a misnomer, since the tea is not processed using a fermenting organism, but oxidized by a process of breaking down the structure of the leaf and exposing it to the air. Green tea is not oxidized; oolong tea is called semi-fermented, which indicates it is oxidized for a short time; and black tea is fully fermented or oxidized. Black and green tea are made from the same types of leaves; it's the processing that makes them taste, smell and look so different.

The most popular teas include green teas such as gunpowder, hyson, dragonwell; oolongs such as Formosa oolong, Ti Kuan Yin, and Wuyi; black teas such as lapsang souchong, yunnan and pu-erh. Blended Chinese black teas include the familiar English and Irish breakfast teas; and scented teas include jasmine, which is made with green tea, and Earl Grey, which combines China black with oil of bergamot.

HOW TO MAKE A PERFECT CUP OF TEA

A perfect cup of tea is made with boiling water and loose tea, steeped for the proper length of time, and then drunk immediately.

1. Rinse the teapot without using soaps or cleaning products.
2. Use filtered or springwater.
3. Black tea should be made by placing leaf tea in the bottom of the pot—one teaspoon per cup—and then pouring water that has been at a full boil directly on the leaves. Steep for four to five minutes.
4. Green tea should be made with water that has barely reached boiling. Steep for three minutes.
5. Oolong teas have hearty, large leaves and should be brewed with water brought to a full boil. You can steep oolong tea for up to ten minutes without it becoming acrid or bitter.

In general, black tea can only be steeped once; some green teas will produce additional cups if water is poured over the damp leaves and they are steeped for one minute. Good-quality oolongs can be reused several times.

CHAPTER SEVEN

Rebuilding the Essential Substances and Organ Systems

Treating Disharmony with Chinese Medicine Dietary Therapy

Treating disharmony with Chinese dietary therapy is the first step in reclaiming wholeness and balance. In some instances, it is the lead medicine in a treatment plan; at other times, it serves as an adjunct to acupuncture and herbal remedies and/or Western therapies, helping the other treatments work more effectively.

THE FIRST-STEP DIETARY THERAPY PROGRAM

Anyone suffering from imbalances (unless they are extremely weak or deficient) can benefit from a program of general detoxification and purification. Dietary therapy gives the body a break—a time to calm down, gather its forces and clear out foods that are causing disharmony or discomfort. This allows for restoration of normal bowel function so the body can harmoniously absorb and utilize food and can harmonize the Qi and the other Essential Substances.

The program is especially helpful to those with digestive troubles such as colitis, lactose intolerance, or irritable bowel syndrome; immune system difficulties such as allergies, hepatitis, HIV, or chronic fatigue; chronic gynecological disturbances; chronic sore throats or colds; and skin disturbances.

GUIDELINES

• The First-Step Dietary Therapy program should be followed within the context of a total healing program under the supervision of a licensed practitioner.

• Each phase may run from one day to one week. You and your practitioner can determine the duration.

• If a phase seems inappropriate for your specific situation, please skip it and go on to the next one.

• Please do not use any phase that may cause weight loss if you are already losing weight due to disease.

• The phases are intended to help you to detoxify as well as rebuild your energy and health. If you feel weak or unable to do a phase, you may skip or shorten it.

Phase One

To tonify the Spleen and Stomach, limit your diet to the following foods for one to seven days.

Miso broth: Miso is a fermented paste made from grains and beans, originating in Japan. It contains bacteria that replenish the flora that may have been depleted or destroyed in the digestive tract through antibiotic or hormone use, poor diet, alcohol intake, or stress. Try using mugi (barley) miso with some mellow yellow (light yellow miso) if it is summertime. Avoid hatcho (dark) except when it is very cold.

Vegetable broth and juices: Fresh organic vegetable broth and juices can be used during this phase. These could include carrot, beet, celery, daikon, watercress, or beet juices. Avoid adding onion or garlic at this stage. When vegetables are juiced, they increase in Yang qualities and may become more warming than just the raw vegetable. It is also much easier to digest raw juice than raw vegetables. We also recommend that you cook the juice into a hot broth as well. You may add an unsalted pure vegetable powder used for vegetable stock to the fresh vegetable broth. This increases the nutrients as well as the flavor.

Lentil broth (cook lentils, strain off the water, and drink the broth as a soup) may also be used in addition to the vegetable broths.

If you have an immune system disorder, all vegetables must be washed thoroughly to avoid parasites. Wash vegetables in a dilute bleach solution (1/2 teaspoon of Clorox bleach in a quart of water) to kill microorganisms. Rinse off the bleach completely after washing.

Brown rice cereal: Brown rice cereal provides added protein and energy. You can find this in any natural food store.

Phase Two

If you have comfortably tried phase one, you may want to move on to phase two for no more than seven days. You also may choose to skip it and go directly to phase three.

Add steamed fresh organic vegetables, especially root vegetables (carrots, daikon root, burdock, beets) and green vegetables (broccoli, kale, chard). Again, make sure all your vegetables are washed thoroughly in a dilute bleach solution, remembering that organic vegetables are grown in manure, which is filled with microorganisms.

Phase Three

Again, use this phase only if you feel strong. Follow this phase for no more than seven days.

Add organic cooked grains, including brown rice, millet, barley, and buckwheat. If you have a very hot condition, avoid buckwheat. Check with your practitioner for advice. You may also add unbleached white rice or white basmati rice for diarrhea. Avoid wheat, corn, and oats. No bread products are included in this phase.

Note: In all three phases, you may use a rice-based protein powder or predigested protein if necessary to prevent weakness and too much weight loss. Don't use milk-based or soy-based protein powder, which may cause diarrhea and produce damp cold.

Phase Four

Add other organic foods and fish. Watch for any unfavorable reactions to foods and eliminate them from your diet, but make sure not to sacrifice balance and sound nutrition.

Phase Five

Once you establish a moderate natural food diet that is unrestricted except by your health considerations, you will have entered phase five, a dietary regime for lifelong good health and harmony.

Tip: If going through phases one to four in order feels too restrictive, you may begin your first-step dietary program with phase four, a generally healthy diet based on organic grains and vegetables with animal protein as an accent. Once you are comfortable with that eating style, you might choose to go back to phase one and try a tonifying routine for one to seven days.

THERAPEUTIC RECIPES

To augment your dietary program, the delicious but medicinal foods presented here will provide you with well-balanced energy and nutrition.

To Purify Xue

KICHAREE
Combine ½ cup cooked mung beans or lentils with ½ cup steamed brown rice. Sauté in sesame oil or clarified butter (ghee) for five minutes with a

pinch of cumin seed, ⅓ teaspoon turmeric, and 1 teaspoon ground coriander.

Then add 4 cups of water and simmer for 20–25 minutes. If desired, this can be topped with a small amount of yogurt.

Kicharee is well balanced and high in easily assimilated protein.

From Abigail Surasky, L.Ac.

To Regain Strength

CONGEE

Rice is often used for healing in Chinese medicine. Congee or rice porridge is an extremely therapeutic food that strengthens the constitution of those who suffer from chronic disease and of those who are convalescing. Many Chinese families eat congee at least once a week to help prevent disharmony.

There are many varieties suitable for different conditions. Your Chinese medicine practitioner can give you recipes using herbs and/or meat and vegetables that are specific for your constitution or diagnosis.

The basic method to make congee is as follows.

Cook 1 cup of rice in 7–9 cups of filtered water for 6–8 hours. A Crock-Pot is extremely useful for simmering congee while you are off doing other things. Traditional Chinese families serve congee made with herbs such as ginseng, Dang Gui, codonopsis, red dates, ginger and ligustrum on a weekly basis. Astragalus is good as an immune tonic congee.

Wheat congee is soothing to the spirit and cooling to fevers.

Sweet rice congee strengthens the Stomach, tonifies Qi and is a tonic for diarrhea and vomiting.

To add additional health-giving properties to congee, use ¼ cup of the following ingredients for every 1–1½ cups of congee.

Mung bean congee cools fevers and aids in detoxification.

Adzuki bean congee removes Dampness, helps ease swelling and edema and aids in treatment of Bladder-Kidney problems.

Carrot congee eases indigestion and dysentery.

Leek or garlic congee warms and tonifies.

Kidney congee is used to tonify the Kidneys and helps with impotence, premature ejaculation and lumbago.

Liver congee helps fight general Yin Deficiencies and strengthens the Liver.

Lamb congee helps rebalance poor circulation and coldness. It is often recommended for women with the addition of ginger and Dang Gui (see herb chapter).

Chicken congee with ginger and Dang Gui added is also good for women.

Beef congee bolsters a weak Spleen and aids those with hypoglycemia.

Qi and Xue Tonics

Chicken Broth Chicken broth is the base of many soups that are used as Xue and Qi tonics in Chinese medicine. Taken plain, it serves as a Xue tonic. When chicken is added, however, it can create congestion and dampness. When possible, use free-range, antibiotic- and hormone-free chicken to make your broth.

This is a secret family recipe.

GRAMMY ETHEL'S CHICKEN BROTH

Place a plump, 3-pound chicken in an 8–10-quart pot of water. Cover, bring to a boil, and then reduce heat to simmer for 1 hour.

Tie 1 parsnip, 1 carrot, and 1 onion in an unbleached cheesecloth bag and immerse in broth.* Cover and cook for another hour.

Remove cheesecloth sack and the whole chicken. Boiled chicken can be eaten separately or added to the broth when appropriate.

Place pot of broth, covered, in refrigerator overnight. The next day, skim fat from top of broth.

Reheat and serve. This nearly fat-free broth can be used alone or as a base for soup or congee. Add rice, vegetables, herbs, or even a nice matzo ball, if you can eat wheat.

CHINESE GINGER CHICKEN SOUP

Remove skin from a 3-pound, whole chicken. Place chicken in a 10-quart pot and cover with water. Bring to a boil, then turn down to a simmer.

Add 5 scallions, sliced lengthwise and then cut in half, to the pot. Cut 1 fresh ginger root in half and slice into slivers about ½ inch long and 1/16 inch wide. Add to pot.

Simmer chicken, scallions and ginger for 1½ hours, covered.

When finished, remove chicken and debone. Return chicken chunks to pot. Add salt to taste if you wish.

DANG GUI CHICKEN

This chicken soup, made with Dang Gui, is good for keeping the Essential Substances and Organ Systems in harmony. If you have one serving a week, you'll find you are stronger and less vulnerable to disease.

You will need a special covered Chinese clay pot—available in Chinatowns and kitchen specialty stores—that resembles an angel food cake or Bundt pan.

Fill a regular 3-quart saucepan with water.

Roll a two-yard length of cheesecloth lengthwise into a long sausage shape and place as a collar along the rim of the saucepan. (When done, rinse for

*Aunt Jane's recipe adds a clove of garlic.

reuse.) Place the clay cooking pot on top of the cheesecloth ring, as if it were the top of a double boiler.

Place one medium chicken, cut up into about 10 pieces, into the clay pot. Add 20 grams of the herb Dang Gui.

You may add ginger and root vegetables such as carrots, turnips, potatoes, onions and parsnips if you like.

Cook over low heat for 1–2 hours until chicken is completely cooked and there is ample broth accumulated in the upper pot. Salt to taste.

Eat one to two servings a week.

For Vitalizing Xue

SAN QI CHICKEN

Prepare this herb recipe in exactly the same way as Dang Gui Chicken, above. Substitute 20 grams of San Qi for the Dang Gui. Eat one to two servings a week to improve circulation.

To Aid Digestion

Miso soup, which rebuilds intestinal flora, is used to rebalance digestion. Its salty flavor can also stimulate the Kidneys.

BASIC MISO SOUP

5 cups water
1 strip kombu, hijiki, or other sea vegetables (You can buy seaweed and the like at many health food stores and Japanese groceries.)
1 cup chard, kale, or other greens
½ cup carrots, sliced
5 teaspoons miso

Rinse kombu or sea vegetable in cold water for 10 minutes. (If using arame, do not soak.) Wipe kombu with dry towel to remove excess sodium. Cut kombu into small strips and add to pot. Bring water to boil. Add carrots. Cover and reduce flame to medium-low. Simmer for about 10 minutes. Take a little of the broth out to mix with miso to form a puree (miso should not be boiled because it will kill the beneficial bacteria). Return miso to the pot and simmer 2 or 3 minutes. Add chard, kale, etc. Simmer 2 minutes.

Serves 4.

HEARTY MISO VEGETABLE SOUP

6 cups water
1 cup hijiki (soaked)
½ cup daikon, diced
½ cup carrots, sliced
1 cup greens (kale, chard, beet tops, etc.)
½ cup cooked brown rice, barley, or beans
1 teaspoon grated ginger or garlic
½ cup green onions, thinly sliced (for garnish)
1 teaspoon sesame oil
6 shiitake mushrooms, sliced (fresh, medium-sized). If you use dried, soak
* overnight and throw out the water.*
6 teaspoons pureed miso (mugi miso)

Soak and rinse sea vegetables. Bring water to a boil and add sea vegetables. Add oil. Reduce to medium-low and simmer 10 minutes. Add carrots and daikon and simmer 3 minutes. Add rice or beans. Add ginger or garlic. Simmer 3 minutes. Add shiitake mushrooms and greens. Simmer three minutes. Serve and garnish with green onions.

Serves 4.

FISH STOCK

1 cup chopped onion
1 cup chopped celery
1 cup chopped carrots
1 lb. fish bones, heads, etc.
3 qts. springwater
1 strip kombu sea vegetable
2 bay leaves
½ teaspoon thyme

Put enough oil in the pot to cover the bottom. Add bay leaves and thyme and simmer vegetables until they become soft. Add fish bones, etc. Stir and simmer. Add water and bring to simmer (do not boil). Add spices and continue to simmer one hour.

Fish stock may be frozen.

WATERCRESS SOUP

5 cups springwater
1 strip kombu, soaked and sliced
4 shiitake mushrooms, sliced
½ cup tofu, cubed into ¼-inch pieces
½ bunch watercress
4 teaspoons mugi miso

Place kombu in water and bring to a boil for 15 minutes. Add shiitake mushrooms and reduce to simmer for 10 minutes. Remove a little of the broth to puree miso. Add tofu and return miso puree to broth. Put a little watercress into each serving bowl and pour the hot soup over. (This is enough to cook the watercress.)

Serves 4 or 5.

THERAPEUTIC VEGETABLES

Eating several vegetables in every meal provides a sound nutritional remedy for many disharmonies. Try to combine one root vegetable, one sea vegetable, one ground vegetable, and one leafy vegetable. For example: daikon and arame and broccoli and chard; carrot and hijiki and snow peas and kale; beets and wakame and acorn squash and bok choy; or onions and arame and cauliflower and mustard greens.

Steam vegetables until cooked but crisp. Sea vegetables, such as seaweed, may need to soak in water for ten to fifteen minutes to become soft enough to steam. Rinsing after soaking will reduce the sodium level up to 50 percent.

Remember to eat vegetables according to the season to take advantage of fresh, local produce. For example, root vegetables are recommended in the winter.

COMMONLY ASKED QUESTIONS ABOUT DIET

Q: Do I have to change how I eat today?

A: No. I would never say you should or shouldn't eat this or that.

For people who have chronic sinusitis, general fatigue or digestive problems, diet therapy is used immediately. But for others, dietary changes can be more gradual.

The guiding principle is that adjustment is more important than radical change.

Embracing Chinese medicine dietary practices is a process of expanding what you eat, not constricting your diet. You may give up some foods, but you should find there's a whole world of varied foods you may have never tried before. To make a shift in your diet—from out of balance to balanced—you must find the place in your heart and consciousness that makes the transition comfortable and unforced.

Discovering the best way for you to improve your diet is a very personal process. You can't rush it—you must give yourself the time to learn about how your body functions and adjust to what it tells you.

Q: Is it better to eat Oriental foods than an American diet?

A: Becoming healthy is not about growing up in Pennsylvania and eating like someone from Beijing. Chinese dietary philosophy suggests that you generally embrace your native foods and eat foods grown locally and in season. What is unhealthy about American foods is not the fact that they are American but that they are too often commercial inventions instead of natural foods. Stick to natural, home-grown, and chemical-free products and you'll have a bountiful supply of healthful food choices.

Q: Is meat bad for you?

A: No, but the body handles meat protein best in small quantities. You should eat no more than two to three ounces at a meal, limit the amount of red meat you eat to about six ounces a week, and begin to think of it as an accent, not the centerpiece in any meal.

Q: What about sugar?

A: Sugar is also part of a balanced diet when eaten in small quantities. Refined sugars have the fewest nutrients, but other sugars such as fructose are contained in nutritionally beneficial foods. Chinese medicine sometimes prescribes sugar as a tonic.

Q: I'm pregnant. Should I change my diet completely?

A: It's not a good idea to make a radical shift in your diet during pregnancy. You want to eliminate coffee, alcohol, drugs and cigarettes. As for other shifts, simply concentrate on eating the most nutrition-packed calories possible. That will naturally lower your fat intake and increase the grains and vegetables.

 If you are planning to become pregnant, however, you may want to make a dietary renovation part of your plan.

 Whatever you do, remember the growing embryo requires fuel. Women who eat too few calories in an attempt to control weight gain or follow some strict food plan are hurting themselves and their baby.

Q: What will happen when I change my diet?

A: A diet rich in grains and legumes, poor in fats and refined sugars can come as a surprise to your body. It will free the Qi to move throughout your system and that can evoke all kinds of transitory negative feelings until the flow is established. That's why you want to go through the process gradually and comfortably. You may want to work simultaneously with other aspects of healing such as herbs and acupuncture since they all reinforce one another.

 If you feel you need to help your body purify itself, you may want to eat Liver cleansing foods such as beets, carrots, and burdock.

Q: Are all grains good for healing?

A: Yes. All of the grains can be used to make healing congees—Chinese therapeutic rice soups (see recipe on page 98). However, some grains are not for everyone. For example, since most Westerners are already too damp and too mucous, I don't recommend oatmeal all that often because in San Francisco I often see people who suffer from Dampness. Oatmeal is beneficial, however, for Lung-Yin Fluid Dryness or Yin Deficiency. Then, if you like, put a little honey, milk and butter on it. This helps increase Yin and fluids.

Q: What can you do to grains to make them appropriate for treating Deficiency or Cold conditions?

A: Add spicy or warm foods such as scallions, ginger, etc. For some of the Spleen Deficiency conditions, a little sweetener is fine. However, honey is contraindicated if you have diarrhea.

Q: What is the most life-extending diet?

A: Chinese medicine has long advocated bland, unprocessed food for a long, healthy life.
Bland food is not flavorless; it is pure and subtle and sweet. Grains, beans, meat and most root vegetables are sweet. We've become used to heavy, overflavored, impure foods that promote dampness, heat, phlegm and a cloudy pallor.

APPLYING DIETARY THERAPY

Dietary therapy provides a powerful tool for correcting disharmonies and is used in conjunction with acupuncture, herbal therapy and Qi Gong to restore balance to the Essential Substances, Organ Systems and channels. Generally, diet therapy can help sedate Excess, tonify Deficiencies, cool off Heat problems, warm up Cold problems, moisten dry problems and dry up Excess Dampness. *Symptoms* describe what you feel when you are not well. *Signs* are the manifestations of disharmony that guide Chinese medicine practitioners when identifying and diagnosing particular imbalances.

TO TREAT DEFICIENT QI

Symptoms include lethargy, loose stools, fatigue, weakness, decreased appetite, shortness of breath, and occasionally, cold extremities and frequent urination.

Signs that your Chinese medicine practitioner will look for include a thin, weak pulse and a tongue that is pale and possibly swollen.

Western diagnoses: Chronic fatigue, asthma, or urinary incontinence.

Your diet should contain the following

Yes. Half of total calories should come from grains and legumes, a third from vegetables, about 15 percent from meats, but to avoid taxing digestion or building mucus, eat only two to three ounces per serving. Five percent of total calories should come from dairy. Recommended foods include rice or barley broth, garlic, leeks, string beans, sunflower seeds, sesame seeds and carrots.

No. Raw food, salads, fruits, and juices in excess.

TO TREAT COLD SYMPTOMS WITH DEFICIENT QI

Eat dried ginger, cinnamon bark, and chicken's eggs. Do not take ginseng without a doctor's advice.

TO TREAT DEFICIENT SPLEEN QI

Symptoms include lack of appetite, bloating, loose stool, and fatigue.

Signs that your Chinese medicine practitioner will look for include a weak pulse and a pale, soft tongue with thin, white fur.

Western diagnoses: diarrhea, gastric or duodenal ulcers, anemia, or even chronic hepatitis.

Your diet should contain the following

Yes. Cooked, warming foods such as squash, carrots, potatoes, yams, rutabagas, turnips, leeks, onions, rice, oats, butter, small amounts of chicken, turkey, mutton or beef, cooked peaches, cherries, strawberries, figs, cardamom, ginger, cinnamon, nutmeg, black pepper, custards, small amounts of honey, molasses, maple syrup and sugar.

Food should be well chewed and eaten in moderate amounts.

No. Salsa, citrus, too much salt, tofu, millet, buckwheat, milk, cheese, seaweed, and excess sugar.

DIETARY GUIDELINES FOR LOOSE STOOLS

For Spleen/Stomach Qi and Yang Deficiencies		*For Food Poisoning*
Digestive tonics:	**Flora-enhancing foods:**	**After sickness subsides . . .**
Warm and cooked foods and moderate-sized meals	Miso	Flora-enhancing foods:
Congees and soups (not cream-based)	Acidophilus	Alfalfa greens
White rice		Kefir
Black tea	**Foods to avoid:**	Miso
Cinnamon tea	Raw and cold foods	Sauerkraut
Barley	Spicy foods	Wheatgrass
Ginger tea	Coffee	Yogurt
	Dairy	**Note:** If loose stools continue, follow Spleen/Stomach Deficiency Guidelines.
	Fats and oils	

TO TREAT DEFICIENT SPLEEN QI LEADING TO DEFICIENT YANG

If Deficient Spleen Qi is not treated early, the body becomes ever more depleted. The Qi cannot be replenished through what you eat and drink. Eventually, a more serious Yang Deficiency develops.

Symptoms include aversion to the cold, a craving for warm drinks, and chilled fingers, toes, ears and nose tip.

Signs that your Chinese medicine practitioner will look for include a slow, thready pulse and a tongue that is moist and pale with indentations on the side.

Western diagnoses: swelling, gastritis, enteritis, kidney disease and colitis.

Your diet should follow the guides for Deficient Spleen Qi, and the following.

No. Raw or chilled foods or those that are hard to digest, such as fatty foods, raw broccoli and milk. They exhaust the digestive fire.

To Treat Dampness Associated with Spleen Qi Deficiency

This is a complicated case of Excess and Deficiency.

Symptoms include headaches, watery stools and queasy stomach.

Signs that your Chinese medicine practitioner will look for include a slippery pulse, tongue fur that is thick and greasy and a tongue body that is swollen with toothmarks along the sides.

Western diagnoses: hepatitis, dysentery, or gastroenteritis.

Your diet should include the same foods that are recommended to treat Deficient Spleen Qi (see page 105) and the following.

Yes. Foods that drain excess dampness such as barley, corn, adzuki beans, garlic, mushrooms, mustard greens, chicken, alfalfa, shrimp, scallions and rye.

No. Too much red meat, salt, or sugar. Also stay away from foods that produce damp, such as dairy, pork, shark meat, eggs, sardines, octopus, coconut milk, cucumber, duck, goose, seaweed, olives, soybeans, tofu, spinach, pine nuts and alcohol.

Dietary Guidelines for Fatigue and Lethargy

Fatigue and Lethargy can stem from Deficiency, Xue Deficiency, Yang Deficiency, Dampness and Qi Stagnation.

To remedy fatigue caused by Qi Deficiency eat foods that tonify Qi and increase energy.

- Cooked and warm foods
- Frequent, small meals
- Sweet foods (not with sugar, but those designated on the food list)
- Cooked, yellow vegetables
- Small amounts of chicken or turkey, especially in soups
- Warming spices such as dried ginger and cinnamon (except with Xue Deficiency)
- Avoid cold or cooling foods and tofu, milk, cheese, and liquids with meals and excess sweet foods

To remedy fatigue caused by Liver Qi Stagnation, eat foods that move Stagnant Qi and motivate stuck energy.

- Chicken livers
- Kelp
- Nori
- Eggplant
- Saffron
- Avoid alcohol, fatty foods, food additives, unnecessary medicines and overindulgence in sweets
- Avoid chicken and turkey
- Spicy foods in small amounts motivate the Qi (see food lists on page 82), but excessive use of spices creates more stagnation.

TO TREAT SPLEEN QI DEFICIENCY WITH DAMP COLD

Symptoms include water retention, puffiness, a cold feeling, mild nausea, trouble breathing, watery stools and clear, frequent urine.

Signs that your Chinese medicine practitioner will look for include a pulse that is weak and slippery or soft and slow and a tongue that is pale with teeth marks on the sides.

Western diagnoses: edema, parasites, ulcers, or Crohn's disease.

Your diet should contain the following

Yes. Grains and legumes equalling 65 percent of total calorie intake. Around a quarter of your diet should be vegetables. Eat only 10 percent red and white meat—no more than twenty-five ounces a week.

No. Raw food, fruits, sugar and dairy products.

TO TREAT SPLEEN QI DEFICIENCY WITH DAMP HEAT

Symptoms include a hot and heavy feeling, fever, nausea, costal or abdominal pain, labored breathing and diarrhea.

Signs that your Chinese medicine practitioner will look for include a weak and slippery or soft pulse that's rapid and a tongue that's swollen and reddish.

Western diagnoses: colitis, acute hepatitis, or Crohn's disease.

Your diet should contain the following

Yes. Grains and legumes equalling 70 percent of calories; cooked vegetables, 30 percent; and white meats, 5 percent—not more than twelve ounces a week. An occasional salad is suggested.

No. Red meat, raw vegetables, fruit juices and dairy products.

TO TREAT UPWARD MOVEMENT OF QI AND MUCUS

This condition is the result of several underlying disharmonies that, only when added together, create symptoms. First, the stresses and strains of daily life coincide with a stressful diet of sugar, caffeine, and alcohol or drugs. This exhausts the Kidney Fire (in the Lower Burner) and digestion (Middle Burner) becomes sluggish. Mucus builds up. Simultaneously, stress triggers an elevation in Liver Yang. Negative emotions make the Liver energy rise upward. Qi and fluid from the Lungs rises and becomes rebellious, uncontrolled, and erratic. This combines with the excess mucus production.

Symptoms include sexual problems, cold extremities, low back pain, susceptibility to every passing cold or flu, joint pain, fear, anxiety and impatience.

Your Chinese medicine practitioner will look for various manifestations, but whatever else is present, there are always the signs of weak Spleen, Kidney and Stomach Systems.

Western diagnoses: sinus allergies, watery eyes, skin rashes, sinus headaches, or chronic cough.

Your diet should include the following

Yes. Cooked foods, rice, mung beans, sweet rice congee, adzuki beans, mustard greens and vegetable broth–based vegetable soups.

No. Sugar, coffee, alcohol, citrus, dairy, soy, all raw, iced, or chilled foods and all energetically cool and cold food.

To Treat Excess Heat

Symptoms include warm or hot extremities, sweatiness, acne or boils, decreased bowel movements, a loud voice, irritability and feeling hot.

Signs that your Chinese medicine practitioner will look for include rapid, full pulse and a tongue that is red and may have a yellow coating.

Western diagnoses: skin disorders accompanied by redness; digestive difficulties; chronic constipation; manic behavior; and/or headaches.

Your diet should contain the following

Yes. Almost half of your total calories should be grains and legumes. A third should be from raw and cooked vegetables. About 20 percent should be from juices and fruits.

No. Frozen or icy foods and chicken. Eat only minimal amounts of meat, sugar and dairy products.

DIETARY GUIDE FOR CONSTIPATION CAUSED BY DRYNESS

Foods That Lubricate Bowels	Foods That Promote Bowel Movement	Flora-Enhancing Foods
Alfalfa sprouts	Asparagus	Alfalfa Greens
Apples	Bran	Kefir
Apricot	Cabbage	Miso
Bananas	Coconut	Sauerkraut
Beets	Fig	Wheatgrass
Carrots	Papaya	Yogurt
Cauliflower	Peas	
Honey	Potato	
Oil		
Okra		
Peaches		
Pears		
Pine nuts		
Prunes		
Seaweed		
Sesame seeds		
Soy products		
Spinach		
Walnut		
Wheat		

To Treat Stagnation of Liver Qi

Symptoms include tenderness in rib cage, nausea, premenstrual lability, irritability and swollen breasts and abdomen.

Signs that your Chinese medicine practitioner will look for include a wiry pulse and a tongue that is dusky or purplish.

Western diagnoses: alcohol abuse, type A personality, fibrocystic breasts, swelling or lumps in groin or breasts, goiter, PMS, menstrual irregularities, or headaches.

Your diet should include the following

Yes. Liver-sedating foods such as beef, chicken livers, celery, kelp, mussels, nori, plums and amazake, a fermented rice drink. Also recommended are foods that regulate or move Qi such as basil, bay leaves, beets, black pepper, cabbage, coconut milk, garlic, ginger, leeks, peaches, scallions and rosemary.

No. Alcohol, coffee, fatty foods, fried foods, excessively spicy foods, heavy red meat, sugar and sweets.

To Treat Fluid Dryness

Symptoms include dry throat, dizziness, emaciation, spontaneous sweating and shortness of breath. Other symptoms vary depending on whether the underlying syndrome is Xue Deficiency or Yin Deficiency.

Signs that your Chinese medicine practitioner will look for include a pulse that is fine, halting, or hollow and weak and a tongue that is uncoated and pink.

Western diagnoses: Type II diabetes or chronic constipation.

Your diet should include the following

Yes. Dairy products, most noncitrus fruits, honey, pork, liver congee, tofu, olive oil, peanut oil and sesame oil. For Kidney Yin Deficiency, eat kidney congee and liver congee. See Xue Deficiency and Yin Deficiency for additional guidelines.

No. Raw fruits and vegetables, cold foods, caffeine, purgative herbs and medicines and alcohol.

To Treat Xue Deficiency

Symptoms include dizziness, low weight, blurred vision, tingling toes or fingers, dry skin or hair and a pale, lusterless face. The symptoms vary depending on the relative Xue Deficiency in a specific Organ System.

Signs that your Chinese medicine practitioner will look for include a thready pulse and a pale tongue.

Western diagnoses: anemia, headaches, anxiety, nervousness and a lack of or painful monthly periods.

Your diet should include the following

Yes. Oysters, sweet rice, liver, chicken soup, Dang Gui Chicken (see recipe on page 99), eggs and green beans.

No. Raw fruit and vegetables, cold liquids and ice.

TO TREAT STAGNANT XUE

Stagnant Xue results from a traumatic injury or as a manifestation of gynecological imbalances.

Symptoms include missed periods, excessive clotting with period, fixed, painful lumps, dry skin and lips, thirst, easily chilled extremities and constipation.

Signs that your Chinese medicine practitioner will look for include a choppy pulse and a tongue that is purple and may have purple spots on the sides.

Western diagnoses: endometriosis, menstrual cramps, PID, fibroids, bruising and fixed pain.

Your diet should include the following

Yes. A small amount of chives, cayenne, eggplant, saffron, safflower, basil, brown sugar and chestnuts to improve Xue circulation.

Turmeric, adzuki beans, rice, spearmint, chives, garlic, vinegar, basil, scallion, leeks, ginger, chestnut, rosemary, cayenne, nutmeg, kohlrabi, eggplant and white pepper to disperse Stagnant Xue.

HOW FIVE PHASES PRACTITIONERS USE DIET THERAPY

Five Phases practitioners put an emphasis on the flavors associated with the phases. When the diet becomes unbalanced, the flavors may become excess or deficient. That can trigger disharmony in associated Organ Systems. To remedy the imbalance, Five Phases diet therapy advocates the addition of counterbalancing flavors, and each has special powers to restore balance.

1. *Wood is associated with sour.* Sour is astringent and gathering. A diet that has an excess of sour is associated with weakening of the Spleen, overproduction of saliva by the Liver and injury to the muscles. It can be counteracted by the addition of metal-pungent foods.

2. *Fire is associated with bitter.* Bitter is drying and strengthening. A diet that has an excess of bitter is associated with Spleen energy dryness, congestion of Stomach energy and a withering of the skin. It can be counteracted by the addition of salty foods.

3. *Earth is associated with sweet.* Sweet is harmonizing and retarding. A diet that has an excess of sweet is associated with achy bones, unbalanced Kidneys, full Heart energy and hair loss. It can be counteracted by the addition of sour foods.

4. *Metal is associated with hot, pungent, aromatic.* Metal is dispersing. A diet that has an excess of pungent is associated with muscle knots, slack pulse, a damaged Shen, and unhealthy fingernails and toenails. It can be counteracted by the addition of bitter foods.

5. *Water is associated with salty.* Salty is softening. A diet that has an excess of salty is associated with deficient muscles and flesh, lack of strength in the large bones and depression. It can be counteracted by the addition of sweet foods.[1]

Rice, trout, small amounts of chicken and chicken liver to strengthen the Stomach/Spleen System to promote sufficient production of Xue.

Mussels, wheat germ, and millet to build Yin, which strengthens Xue.

No. Duck, alcohol, fatty foods and sweets. If you are cold, avoid citrus fruits and tomatoes.

NUTRITIONAL SUPPLEMENTS

Chinese dietary therapy, based on the ancient texts, does not contain suggestions for nutritional supplements. In a perfect world, we wouldn't need them, but food that is contaminated with pesticides, drugs, and hormones, combined with a sedentary lifestyle and constant stress, make it unlikely that most of us receive sufficient nutrition through diet alone.

Using nutritional supplements within the context of Chinese dietary therapy means that you can't substitute vitamin pills for a balanced diet. Popping a pill won't undo the damage done by a low-fiber, high-fat diet. Furthermore, vitamins and minerals are meant to work together and taking too much of one or not enough of another may have a negative impact on how your body can use many vitamins. That's why I believe that vitamins should be taken only after a consultation with a well-informed practitioner or nutritionist.

SUGGESTED SUPPLEMENTATION

Vitamin C

Vitamin C has a cooling nature and moves Qi downward. It is good for people with heat conditions, but if you have very Deficient Spleen Qi or coldness, don't take it as a supplement. The most effective C comes in ascorbate powder form that is then dissolved in water to make a fizzing drink. Start with one or two grams (1,000 to 2,000 mg) of C a day and increase daily until you reach bowel intolerance (diarrhea or severe intestinal gas). Then cut back until you are comfortable. After stabilizing, you may try to build up the dose again. The brand we use in the clinic is C-Salts from Wholesale Nutrition, although there are several good brands. Vitamin C appears to work as an immune enhancer and an antioxidant that fights the ravages of free radicals that have been linked with heart disease and cancer. High doses of vitamin C may cause kidney stones in those who have a predisposition to the disorder. Vitamin C can erode tooth enamel, so it's important to rinse your mouth with clear water after you have taken powdered C. The recommended daily allowance is 60 mg.

Multivitamin, Multimineral Supplement

According to the U.S. Department of Agriculture, two-thirds of Americans fail to get the recommended daily allowance (RDA) of at least one vital nutrient. And those RDAs are low (see chart on page 113). Most supplements supply doses far in excess of RDAs, and ongoing research indicates there are benefits from higher doses of many vitamins. Among the recent findings:

Folic acid and vitamin E offer protection from a wide array of potential health problems from fetal defects to heart disease and menopausal symptoms. Vitamin E tends to be warming: in an oil form it is more warming and damp; in dry form it is less damp and heat promoting. For protective benefits take 400 to 800 IU of vitamin E; and 0.4 mg of folate (folic acid) a day.

Vitamin A helps prevent heart disease and some cancers, but supplements of the vitamin can have unpredictable effects. You receive more effective benefits from increasing your intake of dark, leafy vegetables. New research indicates that it may be a combination of many related nutrients that makes those foods heart-protecting and cancer-blocking. Nutritionists recommend eating the whole food, not the vitamin A extract, to gain all the health benefits. Vitamin A may also be warming and damp, depending on the source of the nutrient.

Another drawback to Vitamin A supplements is that they can be toxic. However, beta-carotene, the precursor of vitamin A, provides the benefits without the danger of toxicity. I recommend 25,000 to 75,000 IU a day of beta carotene.

The newest research indicates that other carotenes, besides beta, are involved in vitamin A's cancer-fighting abilities: alpha, beta-cryptoxanthin, lutein, zeaxanthin, and lycopene. The best greens to eat for a good dose of carotenoids are dandelion, kale, turnip, arugula, spinach, beets, collard greens, and mustard greens. Four ounces of any kind will give you the RDA for vitamin A. Watermelon, tomatoes, carrots, pumpkin, pink grapefruit, oranges and tangerines also contain one or more of these important nutrients.

The minerals in any multivitamin, multimineral supplement should include zinc, magnesium, chromium, selenium and copper. Be careful not to take high doses of trace minerals without the supervision of a trained practitioner or nutritionist.

Calcium/Magnesium

Supplementation of these two minerals in one balanced pill is a good idea for women, those with night leg cramps, people who have bone fractures, and anyone who drinks a lot of caffeine in coffee or colas. The National Institutes of Health recommends 1,000 mg a day of calcium for men and premenopausal women; 1,500 mg for postmenopausal women who are not taking estrogen. Supplements are important because it is so hard to eat enough calcium in a day. For example, that extra glass of skim milk isn't providing you with the calcium you need because your body can absorb only a third of the available calcium in milk, and much of that is lost. Calcium pacifies the Liver and Heart and calms the Shen and decreases Qi Stagnation. Magnesium has a tendency to move Qi downward and so should not be taken as a supplement if you have Deficient Spleen Qi.

To help maintain sufficient calcium levels, in addition to taking a supplement, you should avoid foods that produce calcium loss. The main culprits are those that contain caffeine (including sodas) and foods that have excessive sodium and phosphorus (meat contains phosphoric acid).

Acidophilus

This organism, found in natural yogurt, is used to promote beneficial bacterial growth in the digestive tract and to suppress yeast (candidiasis). It alleviates dampness, especially the nondairy forms of acidophilus. Recommended dose is a quarter to a half a teaspoon three times a day between meals. The best sources are powdered acidophilus such as Natren brand Superdophilus and Karuna's Primadophilus. The acidophilus should be refrigerated and taken with room temperature or lukewarm water.

THE GOVERNMENT'S RDAs	
Vitamin C	60 mg
B_1 (thiamine)	1.5 mg
B_2 (riboflavin)	1.7 mg
B_3 (niacin)	20 mg
Calcium	800 mg
Iron	18 mg
Vitamin D	400 IU
Vitamin E	30 IU
Biotin	0.3 mg
B_6	2 mg
Folic acid	0.4 mg
B_{12}	6 mcg
Phosphorus	1 g
Iodine	150 mcg
Magnesium	400 mg
Zinc	5 mg
Copper	2 mg
Pantothenic acid	10 mg

Garlic Capsules or Pills

Garlic is very warming and those with heat conditions should avoid eating it. However, it can help reduce fungal infections and has been reported to benefit cardiovascular health. Processed garlic provides the active ingredient your body can use—without the smell or taste.

Essential Fatty Acids

Unprocessed or cold-pressed oils such as linseed, walnut, soy, wheat germ, chestnut, soybean and evening primrose, and fish oils such as salmon, mackerel, cod, haddock and cod liver, influence the various hormones called prostaglandins. These hormones have a counterregulatory relationship: some cause smooth muscle relaxation, some cause smooth muscle contraction; some ease inflammation, some cause inflammation; some decrease blood clotting, some increase clotting. Since our nutritionally deprived diets tend to strengthen the detrimental prostaglandins, we need to take essential fatty acid supplements to give the good prostaglandins a chance to exert their balancing influence.

When taking the oil supplements, keep them refrigerated to prevent them from becoming rancid, and alternate one tablespoon daily of any of the essential fatty acid oils mentioned above.

CHAPTER EIGHT

Dancing with Dang Gui and Friends

A Survey of Chinese Herbal Therapy

Wholeness = Dietary Guidelines + **Herbs** + Acupuncture + Qi Gong

In 3,500 B.C., Shen Nung, the god of husbandry, founded Chinese herbal medicine. According to a tale passed down through the ages, he had a hole in his stomach through which he watched his internal processes. Because of this remarkable ability, he became curious about what happened to his body when he ate various plants, minerals and animals. This led him to take 365 types of herbs in order to determine their healing effects. But even a God could not dodge the perils of experimentation with unknown herbs. After cataloging hundreds of them, he died of poisoning.

The moral of the story—and one that I hope you'll take to heart—is that you should never take any herbs not included in the medicine cabinet section (page 209) without consulting a trained herbalist.

CHARACTERISTICS OF CHINESE HERBAL MEDICINE

Herbs have the power to restore balance to the channels, Organ Systems and Essential Substances. The art and science of using these powerful botanicals, minerals and animal products comes in knowing how to prescribe the right herb or mixture of herbs to do the job.

The process usually begins with a diagnosis of the disharmony. Then the herbalist prescribes an herb or a combination of herbs, depending on how they act, to remedy the problem. There are four ways herbs wield their curative powers: through temperature, taste, direction and organs entered.

***Temperature* is broken down into** Hot, Cold, Warm, Cool and Neutral. If a disease is considered Hot, then an herb with cooling properties is selected. If the disease is considered Cold, then a warming herb is used. The degree of warming and cooling needed will direct the practitioner toward various herbs and combinations of herbs.

Tastes **are characterized as** *Acrid, Sweet, Bitter, Sour* and *Salty.* Taste has an important influence on the therapeutic effect of any herb or combination of herbs. Acrid substances disperse and move; sweet substances tonify and harmonize; bitter substances drain and dry; sour substances are astringent and prevent or reverse the normal leakage of fluids and energy; salty substances purge; and bland substances—that is, those that have no recognized flavor quality—take out dampness and promote urination.

Direction **means that** the energy of herbs rises and floats (moves upward and outward) or falls and sinks (moves downward and inward). The direction of an herb is employed to move Qi and other Essential Substances as required to reestablish harmony. For example, if you suffer from Stagnant Stomach Qi and are suffering from what is diagnosed as Food Stuck in the Stomach, you might use an herb that has downward energy. Or for sinus blockage, you might use an herb with energy that moves upward and helps direct the other herbs in the formula toward the problem.

Organs entered indicates which specific Organ System(s) the herb is able to affect.

FORMS OF HERBAL REMEDIES

Chinese herbs come in many forms, some of which are bulk herbs, powders, pills, tinctures, and decoctions. The two most common forms are bulk herbs and pills. **Bulk herbs** are generally processed before they are used in herbal therapy. They may be altered in order to detoxify substances that would otherwise be harmful or to make the herb more Yang or more cooling or change its energetics so that its tonic effects come to the front. This is done, for example, by baking, dipping in honey, boiling, soaking, or frying the substance before it is turned into powders and decoctions.

Decoctions are made by cooking a combination of prepared bulk herbs in water to make an herb tea or soup. They are useful because, unlike pills, they can be individualized. Decoctions are particularly effective against acute problems such as the External Pernicious Influence Wind-Cold. They are usually not prescribed for more than a few days; if the herbs are required for chronic conditions, many practitioners will provide pills or powders.

Decoctions are also used for steaming, making poultices and other external applications. Not all herbs should be made into decoctions, however. Some, such as ganoderma, which is in many immune-enhancing formulas, lose much or all of their effectiveness when decocted without first being ground into an extremely fine powder.

Powders are usually created by pulverizing one or more herbs to create a formula.

Like a pill, powders are commonly swallowed with warm water. Sometimes they are put into boiling water in a thermos and steeped overnight to create a tea. At other times, practitioners will buy prepared powders or granules that are generally made from decoctions of herbs that have been spray-dried.

TIP

You can tell what form an herb will come in by its name. If it includes the word *tang*, it will be a decoction. *San* means it is a powder. *Wan* or *pien* indicates it is a pill.

Herbal pills almost always contain formulas, not individual herbs, and are targeted to treat specific disharmonies. There are many types of herbal pills—some are made from powders, some from concentrates. They are often favored over bulk herbs because:

1. The cost is lower. Many of the herbs in the formulas are expensive to buy individually, but when purchased in large quantities by the manufacturers of the pills, the cost goes down.
2. They're easier to use. People are more apt to follow the recommended therapeutic routine.
3. They are formulated for specific disharmonies. Some herbal formulas now on the market have been devised to address extremely specific problems and offer the practitioner and patient the assurance of high-quality therapy.
4. Pills have a more concentrated pharmacological effect. (Buy your herbal pills from companies that prepare the herbs in a traditional way, such as frying in honey or cooking in rice wine, before grinding them up. Your physician should ask the herb company how the herbs are prepared.)
5. They provide access to rare or very expensive herbs not carried by most herbal stores, practitioners, or pharmacies.

Internal unguents are prepared by boiling herbs over and over again. The resulting solution is condensed and thickened into a salve and sugar or honey is added to it. External unguents are made by boiling herbs in oil and adding cinnabar and vinegar. The resulting salve is heated and spread over a cloth that is used as a compress or plaster.

Pellets are usually made from extremely rare medicinals and are super-refined into a fine powder that is mixed with a gluey substance. Pellets are used internally and externally.

Elixirs are therapeutic beverages made by soaking or simmering herbs in wine.

Essence is liquid distilled from fresh herbs, and it is for drinking. Essences are usually taken in the summer.

Tinctures or extracts are drinks made by steeping herbs in alcohol or glycerin.

Enemas, made from easily dissolved herbs or cooked teas, are used to remedy digestive problems.

HOW TO PREPARE HERBS AT HOME

If you are given bulk herbs, there are several steps to follow.

1. Boil herbs in clay or glass. Metal cookware can destroy or reduce the effectiveness of the herb. To prepare your clay pot, immerse it in warm water for at least thirty minutes. Allow it to dry completely. Rub all unglazed surfaces with an organic cooking oil. Allow the oiled pot to sit overnight. Wash the pot with warm water; don't ever use soaps or household cleansers on the clay. Re-oil periodically.
2. Place the herbs in the pot and soak the herbs as prescribed by the herbalist.
3. Add enough water to cover the herbs and bring it to a boil, briefly. Turn down to simmer, uncovered. Reduce the liquid as directed.
4. Pour off the liquid and leave the herbs in the pot. Take the infusion as prescribed. Store remaining tea in the refrigerator.
5. The next day, add more water as directed by your practitioner. Repeat steps 3 and 4. Discard the herbs after two days.

COMBINING HERBS

Whatever form the herbs come in, they are often assembled into formulas that combine two or more herbs to produce a targeted effect. The herbs each have one or more roles within the formula. The basic roles are described as:

The chief herb, which is the main active ingredient in the formula.

The deputy herb, which augments or promotes the action of the chief herb or addresses a different pattern of disharmony.

The assistant herb, which reduces side effects or potential toxicity of the chief herb or reinforces the chief herb.

The envoy herb harmonizes the herbs, allowing them to work together as a unit. It can also help focus the herbal activity on a specific area. (Licorice is often used in this capacity.)[1]

The herbs in a formula interact with one another in several ways. They are:

Additive: When two or more herbs with the same effect are used together, their action may be amplified. No herbalist would ever combine herbs without knowing the additive effects.

Synergistic: Sometimes combining two or more herbs produces an effect that is greater than the sum of its parts. When this happens, the herbs are said to potentiate each other.

Mutually restraining: Sometimes two or more herbs are used together to weaken or neutralize some aspect of one or both herbs. This is particularly useful if an herb causes several physiological reactions, only one of which is appropriate for the diagnosis.

Inhibitive: One herb's effect inhibits the action of another herb.

Destructive: The combination of two herbs decreases the toxicity of one.

Oppositional: Opposing herbs are two or more botanicals that are harmful when taken together.

CHOOSING A QUALIFIED HERBALIST

Herbal remedies should be prescribed only by a competent, trained herbalist. Taking recommendations from untrained personnel at health food stores, through mail order catalogs, or from untutored practitioners is foolish at best and dangerous at worst.

In my clinic, I try to use herbal companies that sell only to licensed, primary health care providers or licensed pharmacies. Consumers should beware of herb suppliers who make claims for formulas and then sell to anyone who asks for them.

Although there is no licensing of herbalists, the National Commission for the Certification of Acupuncturists does provide a certificate of training. If you go to a Chinese herbalist who has been dispensing herbs for years, rely on personal recommendations and reputation.

SIDE-EFFECTS OF HERBS

There are some undesirable side effects from herbs and formulas, the most common of which are digestive problems. They usually pass after two to three days, as the body adjusts to increased fiber intake and begins to rebalance itself.

If the side effects persist, they can be controlled by changing the time of day the herbs are taken and the dosage. Sometimes a digestive formula needs to be added to the herbal regimen to restore balance. A practitioner can tell the difference between the presence of a disease that causes digestive upset and herbal side effects.

AN HERB SAMPLER

The following individual herbs are listed in alphabetical order. They are a sampling of the herbal remedies that I prescribe extensively in my clinic and that are commonly used in most Traditional Chinese Medicine practices. At the end of each section are examples of the variety of formulas that use these herbs. I developed Enhance™, Tremella American Ginseng™, Source Qi™, Clear Heat™, Marrow Plus™ and Channel Flow™. These formulas are available from Health Concerns (see resource section) through your local practitioner.

ASTRAGALUS

Astragalus membranaceus (Huang Qi) is one of the most important tonic herbs and is a major ingredient in many formulas to strengthen the Qi. It targets Spleen Qi and increases overall energy, aids in digestion and absorption of food and helps heal injured tissue. Its main chemical constituents have been identified as plant pigments, sugars and acids.

Uses

- For prevention of the common cold[2]
- To build resistance to viruses and bacteria[3]
- To treat chronic kidney inflammation (nephritis) and decrease edema and protein in the urine[4]

According to Western research, astragalus has immune restoration capabilities. Several Chinese studies found it increases the red blood cell count and also claimed increased survival rates in people with lung and liver cancer from 28 percent to 71 percent.[5] In another Chinese study of chronic active hepatitis, liver functions returned to normal in eighteen of thirty-one participants.[6] Animal studies have shown its effectiveness in lowering blood pressure.[7]

Formulas

Bu Zhong Yi Qi Tang (Central Qi Tea)—a Qi tonic

Enhance™—for immune modulation

ATRACTYLODES

Atractylodes alba or white atractylodes (Bai Zhu) is also a Qi tonic. It tonifies the Spleen and Stomach, helps with digestion, and removes dampness. Its chemical constituents are atractylone, actractylol, and vitamin A.[8]

There are many reports from China on the ability of atractylodes to increase white blood cell counts and it is used regularly in formulas for immune enhancement.[9] It also lowers blood sugar and prevents concentration of glycogen in the liver.[10] For cardiovascular disease, it reduces platelet aggregation.[11] This may make it an herb that should be carefully used in idiopathic thrombocytopenia (ITP), a diminution in blood platelet count.

Uses

- To reduce edema
- To increase body weight and muscle strength

Formulas

Central Chi Tea (Bu Zhong Yi Qi Tang) and **Four Gentleman** (Si Jun Zi Tang)—for Qi tonics

Enhance™—for immune modulation

Source Qi™—for Deficient Spleen Yang chronic diarrhea

BUPLEURUM

Bupleurum root (Chai Hu) is what is called a release exterior herb—it is used to treat diseases that cannot be categorized as either interior or exterior, but that are in the process of moving inward. This stage of illness is called Shao Yang (see the six stages of disease) and is associated with pain in the rib cage, alternating chills and fever, a bitter taste in the mouth, and vomiting.

Bupleurum is also used to spread the Liver Qi, allowing the Qi to move more smoothly throughout the body, and to raise the Spleen Qi in order to harmonize Spleen and Stomach deficiency patterns.

Research has revealed that bupleurum has an anti-inflammatory, antiviral, anti-bacterial,[12] and liver-protective effects.[13] Of particular interest are its antibacterial effect against *Mycobacterium tuberculosis* and, in the laboratory, its antiviral effect against influenza and polio viruses.[14] It's often used to lower fevers associated with upper respiratory infections and in Asia, it's used to treat malaria. Its main chemical constituents have been identified as bupleurumol, saponin, phytosterol, adonitol, angelicin and various acids.[15]

Uses

- To reduce fever
- To calm or tranquilize

Formulas

Xiao Chai Hu Tang—for chronic viral infection, particularly CFIDS and hep-atitis

Xiao Yao San—for such disparate Western disorders as chronic hepatitis, pre-menstrual syndrome, and depression

Bu Zhong Yi Qi Tang (Central Qi Tea)—as a Qi tonic and to help with diarrhea and raise the Qi

Ease Plus™—for drug detoxification and anxiety disorder: based on the tra-ditional formula **Bupleurum and Dragon Bone**

CODONOPSIS

Codonopsis (Dang Shen) strengthens and harmonizes the functions of the Spleen and Stomach. It is often used in formulas in the place of Ginseng to increase Qi, especially in persons over the age of forty.

Codonopsis has been shown in Chinese studies to increase red blood cells and to enhance T cell transformation. In combination with other herbs, it increases white blood cell counts in people undergoing chemotherapy and radiation. Chronic kidney disease (nephritis) and anemia are also treated with the herb.

Uses

- To help overcome lack of appetite and fatigue
- To strengthen tired limbs
- To stop vomiting and diarrhea
- To overcome shortness of breath and chronic sputum-producing cough
- To calm the nervous system
- To aid digestion

Formulas

Eight Precious Pills—for tonifying Qi and Xue

Women's Precious Pills (Ba Zhen Tang)—for tonifying Qi and Xue

Shen Ling Qi Bai Zhu Tang—for improving digestion

Source Qi™—for Deficient Spleen Yang chronic diarrhea

DANG GUI

Dan Gui *(radix angelica sinensis)* tonifies the blood and regulates the menses. It also disperses cold. The literal translation means "state of return."

Uses

- To regulate menstruation and ease menstrual pain
- To ease blurred vision
- To moisten dry stools
- To treat abdominal pain and traumatic injury

Formulas

Woman's Balance™

Xiao Yao San

ECLIPTA

Eclipta prostrata (Han Lian Cao) protects the Liver and Kidney Yin. It also cools Xue. Historically, it was used to treat ringing in the ears, premature graying of the hair and to stop bleeding.

Uses

- As a liver-protecting compound for people with hepatitis and liver disease caused by exposure to chemical toxins[16]
- To treat diphtheria, when used with other supportive therapy

Formulas

Ecliptex™—for chronic viral hepatitis, environmental liver contamination and environmental illness (EI)—if herbs can be tolerated

GANODERMA

Ganoderma (Ling Zhi) is a Qi tonic that also tonifies the Xue. There are six types of ganoderma mushrooms, each a different color. The red Ling Zhi is considered the most powerful.[17]

The active ingredients—polysaccharides—are found mostly in the spores. Polysaccharides have a regulatory effect on the immune system.[18] They also contain ergosterol, coumarin, mannitol, polysaccharides, and organic acids.[19]

Uses

- To reduce symptoms in hepatitis[20] and protect the liver from damage,[21] as well as decrease SGPT (a liver enzyme measuring liver function) levels[22]
- To modulate the immune system, particularly in relation to cancer.[23]
- To increase pulmonary function, particularly for asthmatics
- To decrease insomnia—known in Chinese medicine as a calm spirit effect.[24]

Formulas

Enhance™—for immune modulation

Tremella American Ginseng™—for immune modulation

GINSENG

Ginseng (*Panax schinseng*) is a slightly bitter root that is used because it tonifies the spleen and lung, promotes secretion of bodily fluids, replenishes vital energy, and is a sedative. It exerts an effect on the central nervous system; acts as an antihistamine; impacts the endocrine system, including stimulation of brain function; affects the metabolism, including reduction of blood sugar and blood cholesterol; aids as a cardiac tonic, although a large dose can be toxic; and works as an immune enhancer. Its chemical constituents include panaxosides, essential oil, saponin, protopanaxadiol, and protopanaxatriol.[25] Ginseng should not be used by someone with Excess Heat and pathogenic factors.

Uses

- For shock and prostration
- To ease diarrhea and loss of appetite due to Spleen Deficiency
- Dehydration, diabetes
- Palpitation, insomnia, forgetfulness
- Fatigue, extreme weakness

Formulas

Bu Zhong Yi Qi Wan
Source Qi™

AMERICAN GINSENG

American ginseng (*Panax quinquefolius*) is quite distinct from ginseng. It replenishes the Yin, reduces internal heat, and promotes the secretion of bodily fluids. It has been demonstrated to have a sedative effect on the brains of animals in lab experiments, creates an excitatory action on the central nervous system, and is a cardiotonic. Its chemical constituents are panaquilon, panax-sapogenol, oleanolic acid, panacene, phytosterin, sugar, mucilage, and resin.[26] It is contraindicated for anyone with Cold and Damp Stomach symptoms.

Uses

- Chronic cough due to Lung deficiency
- Low-grade fever (usually in the afternoon)
- Spontaneous night sweating
- Fatigue due to chronic consumptive disease

Formulas

Tremella American Ginseng™

ISATIS

Isatis leaf (Da Qing Ye) and isatis root (Ban Lan Gen) are what Chinese medicine calls Clear Heat, Clean Toxin (antiviral, antibacterial) herbs. Isatis root is a major herb used in anticancer formulas in China as well as in treating chronic myelogenous leukemia.[27]

Uses

- To combat viral hepatitis, herpes, and viral meningitis[28]
- To treat pneumonia, meningitis, and erysipelas
- To fight bacterial infections such as shigella, salmonella, streptococcus and staphylococcus.

Formulas

Enhance™—immune modulation

Tremella American Ginseng™—immune modulation

Clear Heat™—for Toxic Heat and viral and bacterial infections

Isatis Gold ™—for External Pernicious Heat with viral symptoms

LICORICE ROOT

Glycyrrhiza glabra or licorice root (Gan Cao) is included in many Chinese herbal formulas in order to allow the various herbs to enter fully all the major channels of the body. For this reason, it is one of the most commonly used herbs in formulas. In addition, it both tonifies the Qi and removes toxins. By itself, it's a Qi tonic and is traditionally used to strengthen the Spleen and help remedy weak digestion.

Japanese and Chinese researchers have explored its anticancer,[29] anti-HIV,[30] antiviral, hepatitis,[31] and anticandida[32] properties. In Germany, a multicenter study with a licorice extract showed a success rate of 30 to 40 percent against chronic viral hepatitis B.[33] It stops pain and spasms, has antitoxicity effect, and is often used as an anti-inflammatory for arthritis and gastric ulcers.

WARNING

In prolonged high doses, *Glycyrrhiza* can be toxic, causing high blood pressure and water retention, reduction in thyroid function, and a decrease in the basal metabolic rate. When mixed properly in an herbal formula, very little is used. Always take *Glycyrrhiza* under the care of a qualified, licensed health care provider.

Uses

- To treat gastric ulcers
- To ease sore throats
- To bolster immunity

Formulas

Four Gentlemen Decoction (Si Jun Zi Tang)—for a Qi tonic

Enhance™—immune modulation

Tremella American Ginseng™—immune modulation

Source Qi™—to counter Deficient Spleen Yang diarrhea

LIGUSTRUM

Ligustrum lucidum (Nu Zhen Zi) is a fruit used to strengthen the Kidney, especially the Kidney Jing and Yin.[34] Such Kidney Tonics are especially effective as immune enhancers,[35] and increase the white blood cell count, especially important in people with HIV/AIDS and people with many forms of cancer. It also acts as a tonic for people who are debilitated and wasting away.

Older people or those who are weak may eat ligustrum in congee.[36] It has broad-spectrum antibacterial effects. The main chemical constituents are oleanolic acid, oleic acid, linoleic acid, fructose, glucose, and mannitol.[37]

Uses

- To ease dizziness and control floating spots in the visual field
- To treat early stages of cataracts
- To ease low back pain
- To stop ringing in the ears
- To lower fever from tuberculosis

Formulas

Enhance™—immune modulation

Er Zhi Wan—tonifies Liver and Kidney Yin, often used to relieve menopausal symptoms

MILLETIA

Milletia reticulata or caulis milletia (Ji Xue Teng) vitalizes and tonifies Xue. Its active ingredient has been identified as milletol.[38]

WARNING

Milletia increases contractions in the uterus, so it's contraindicated during pregnancy unless specifically okayed by a Chinese herbalist and your Western doctor.

Uses

In cancer therapy, milletia stimulates bone marrow function in people undergoing chemotherapy and radiation. It ameliorates the side effects of lowered white blood cell counts and aplastic anemia.[39]

Formulas

Marrow Plus™—to increase bone marrow function

Enhance™—to increase bone marrow function

Tremella American Ginseng™—to increase bone marrow function

SAN QI

San Qi is used for injuries of all types, to disperse Xue and Qi. In combination with other herbs, it is used for pain relief. It should not be taken during pregnancy or if there is profuse bleeding.

Uses

- For treatment of injuries
- Thrombosis
- Postpartum difficulties related to Stagnant Qi and Xue

Formulas

San Qi 17™—to relieve pain, treat injuries and problems related to Stagnant Xue

Xiong Dan Die Da Wan—for trauma and injuries

Jin Gu Shang Wan—for trauma and injuries

Tang-kuei and Lindera Formula—for postpartum difficulties

SCHIZANDRA

Chinese traditional medicine categorizes the schizandra fruit (Wu Wei Zi) as an astringent, a Qi tonic and a Kidney tonic, good for calming the spirit and increasing memory functions. Its active ingredients have been identified as essential oils, lignans, citric acid, ascorbic acid and fumaric acid

This herb is particularly effective in treating Western liver disease: In a Chinese study, schizandra showed effectiveness in lowering SGPT (liver enzyme) levels in 72 percent of 102 patients over an average period of twenty-five days.[40] It also acts as an astringent to the intestines.

Uses

- To increase brain function
- To decrease insomnia
- To stop asthmatic breathing (when used in formulas)
- To ease diarrhea and urinary problems (when used in formulas)
- To stop excessive night or day sweats

Formulas

Schizandra Dreams™—for insomnia

Tian Wang Bu Xin Wang—for insomnia

Enhance™—immune modulation

Tremella American Ginseng™—immune regulation with Yin Deficiency

Ecliptex™—for protection of the Liver

VIOLA

Viola yedoensis (Zi Hua Di Ding) is a Clear Heat Clean Toxin herb and is used often in formulas for persons suffering from viral or bacterial infection. Its identified chemical constituents are cerotic acid and saponin.

Viola deserves special mention here because it was the most potent antiviral agent when tested in vitro during research on HIV at the University of California at Davis and Hong Kong University.[41] It was also suggested by the World Health Organization in 1989 for study as a cost-effective antiviral agent against HIV.[42] It is a common component of anticancer formulas in China.

In addition, viola has antibacterial properties, particularly against streptococcus, pseudomonas[43] and mycobacterium.[44]

Uses

- To counter bacterial infections such as carbuncles and deep furuncles
- For malignant lesions
- Scrofula

Formulas

Enhance™—immune modulation

Tremella American Ginseng™—immune modulation with Yin Deficiency

Clear Heat™—for Clear Heat Clean Toxin effects on HIV and other viruses

SILYBUM

Silybum marianum or milk thistle is a Western herb that has long been used in Europe for the treatment of liver disorders.[45,46] Silybum has been shown to stimulate liver cell proteins, leading to more rapid recovery of liver cells after they are damaged.[47] It has also shown positive effects on gastric ulceration in a study in rats.[48] Results from a Hungarian study indicate that silymarin (an extract of Silybum) is able to increase antioxidant protection in cells.[49] Silybum's chemical constituents have been identified as silymarin and flavolignans.[50]

Uses

- To protect the liver
- As an antioxidant
- To lower liver enzymes and decrease liver damage in persons with chronic viral hepatitis and chemical damage to the liver

Formulas

Ecliptex™—for chronic viral hepatitis. I generally use it in conjunction with an immunomodulatory formula such as **Enhance**™ or **Tremella American Ginseng**™ because there is some basis for suspecting that chronic viral hepatitis is also an immune dysfunction disorder.

Herb	Chinese Description	Properties	Current Use	Sample Formulas
American ginseng	Benefits Qi Tonifies Yin Generates Jin-Ye	Reduces internal heat Promotes secretion of bodily fluids Cardiotonic	Chronic cough Low-grade fever Fatigue	Tremella American Ginseng™
Astragalus (Huang Qi)	Qi tonic Spleen tonic	Immune restoration Anticancer Antibacterial Antiviral	General immune tonic To resist colds & flu Prolapses	Enhance™ Source Qi™ Tremella American Ginseng™ Astra Isatis™ Central Chi Tea
Atractylodes (Bai Zhu)	Qi tonic Spleen/Stomach tonic	Immune enhancement Increase white blood cell count Liver glycogen	Body weight Muscle strength Diarrhea	Enhance™ Source Qi™ Central Chi Tea

Herb	Chinese Description	Properties	Current Use	Sample Formulas
Bupleurum (Chai Hu)	Releases exterior Spreads Liver Qi Spleen tonic	Protects liver	Antiviral Antibacterial Anti-inflammatory Hepatitis Upper respiratory infections PMS	Xiao Chai Hu Tang Central Chi Tea Xiao Yao San Ease Plus™
Codonopsis (Dang Shen)	Harmonizes Spleen and Stomach	Enhances T cell transformation Increases red blood cell count	Immune tonic Cancer support Appetite	Source Qi™ Eight Precious Pills
Dang Gui	Disperses Cold Tonifies Xue	Regulates blood Reduces Thrombosis	Menstrual irregularities and pain Dry stools Abdominal pain	Woman's Balance™ Xiao Yao San
Eclipta (Han Lian Cao)	Yin tonic Cool Xue	Stop bleeding Protect liver	Hepatitis Liver damage	Ecliptex™
Ganoderma (Ling Zhi)	Qi tonic	Immunomodulation Liver enzymes Anticancer	General immune tonic HIV/AIDS CFIDS Viral hepatitis	Enhance™ Resist™ Tremella American Ginseng™ Bioherb™
Ginseng	Tonifies Yuan Qi Strengthens Spleen and Stomach Calms Shen	Regulates blood sugar Increases appetite Increases heart contractions Increases immune response	Diarrhea Loss of appetite Insomnia Memory lapses	Bu Zhong Yi Qi Wan Source Qi™
Isatis (Da Qing Ye and Ban Lan Gen)	Clear Heat Clean Toxin	Antiviral Antibacteria Anticancer	Herpes Colds and flu Viral hepatitis Viral meningitis	Enhance™ Tremella American Ginseng™ Clear Heat™
Licorice (Gan Cao)	Harmonizes Qi tonic Removes toxins	Anticancer Antiviral Anticandida Anti-inflammatory	Immune tonic Gastric ulcers Sore throat	Enhance™ Tremella American Ginseng™ Four Gentlemen Source Qi™

Herb	Chinese Description	Properties	Current Use	Sample Formulas
Ligustrum (Nu Zhen Zi)	Kidney tonic Yin tonic	Immune modulation	Immune tonic Retinitis Early graying Increase white blood cell count	Enhance™ Tremella American Ginseng™
Milletia (Ji Xue Teng)	Xue tonic Xue vitalizer	Bone marrow function	Anemia Cancer support	Enhance™ Tremella American Ginseng™ Marrow Plus™
San Qi	Qi and Xue tonic	Pain relief Dispel blood clots	Treat injuries Manage post-partum circulatory problems	San Qi 17™ Xiong Dan Die Da Wan Jin Gu Shang Wan Tang-kuei and Lindera Formula
Schizandra (Wu Wei Zi)	Kidney tonic Qi tonic	Liver enzymes Brain function	Insomnia Diarrhea Excess sweating Hepatitis	Schizandra Dreams™ Tremella American Ginseng™ Enhance™ Ecliptex™
Silybum (milk thistle)	Not cataloged	Immunomodulation Protects liver Antioxidant	Hepatitis Liver damage	Ecliptex™
Viola (Zi Hua Di Ding)	Clear Heat Clean Toxin	Antiviral Antibacterial Anticancer	HIV Boils Carbuncles	Enhance™ Tremella American Ginseng™ Clear Heat™

COMMONLY MISUSED HERBS

There are several herbs that are often misused and may cause significant health problems if self-prescribed.

Echinacea and goldenseal are often taken by people with chronic viral illnesses. These two herbs are meant to be used for acute, not chronic, viral illnesses—at the beginning of a cold or flu, for example. Furthermore, studies show that echinacea increases tumor necrosis factor (TNF)[51], so long-term, high-dose use may weaken rather than strengthen the immune system. Also, goldenseal can be toxic when taken for too long, since it is stored in the liver and not excreted.

There are many formulas found in health food stores using the combination of echinacea and goldenseal. They should only be used when you are trying to relieve a cold or flu or acute viral symptoms. Better yet, consult a practitioner to prescribe Chinese or Western herbs that are specific to your condition.

Another commonly misused herb is ephedra or Ma Huang. Ma Huang is used in Chinese formulas for lung disease, acute viral illness (External Wind Invading the Surface), and, especially, asthmatic breathing. Many people can't tolerate Ma Huang because it has ephedrine in it, which speeds up the metabolism. Unfortunately, unscrupulous herb manufacturers often put large amounts of ephedra in formulas for weight loss without balancing its effect. Long-term use creates dryness and Yang Excess imbalances. Ma Huang is also contraindicated for people with high blood pressure.

Ginseng (Ren Shen) is used frequently by itself as a general energy tonic. However, it is only indicated when lack of energy is associated with Qi Deficiency. If the problem is Stagnant Qi, it may only worsen the problem. For people over forty, using Chinese or Korean ginseng straight—without combining it with other herbs—can deplete the Yin and warm and tonify the Yang too much. However, American ginseng, which has more Yin tonic effects, is often used. Because of these nuances, it is important to consult a trained Chinese herbalist before taking ginseng—or any Chinese herbs.

CHAPTER NINE

Metal and Fire

The Arts of Acupuncture and Moxibustion

Wholeness = Dietary Guidelines + Herbs + **Acupuncture** + Qi Gong

Acupuncture is the art and science of manipulating the flow of Qi and Xue through the body's channels—the invisible aqueduct system that transports the Essential Substances to the Organ Systems, tissues, and bones. Manipulation of the Qi and Xue is accomplished by the stimulation of specific acupuncture points along the channels where the Essential Substances flow close to the skin's surface.

Present-day practitioners use many different methods for stimulating acupuncture points, including electrostimulation and lasers as well as the traditional fine metal needles. Whatever the technique, acupuncture is relatively painless and often accompanied by feelings of heaviness or warmth and the movement of energy. Such sensations occur because acupuncture points are equivalent to valves in an aqueduct system. When the points are stimulated, they may open a valve, so that Excess or Stagnant Qi or Xue can disperse. If Qi and Xue are Deficient, stimulation of certain acu-points may close a valve, so the Essential Substances can collect as needed. When this is done, the distribution of Essential Substances throughout the whole system of channels becomes more evenly balanced, allowing for a smoother flow into all areas of the body.

This adjustment of the body's Qi and Xue can be used to maintain or restore balance between Yin and Yang, alleviate emotional disorders, protect the Organ Systems, moisten tendons and keep the joints healthy. Acupuncture works on a spiritual level and a physical, energetic level.

TYPES OF ACUPUNCTURE

When it comes time to select an acupuncturist, you may be surprised to find out that there are many different types of practitioners. Some are Traditional Chinese Medicine acupuncturists, as I am; others are Japanese, Korean constitutional, Five

In 1987, George came for treatment for alcoholism and, as he says, "Once I had the acupuncture treatment, I stopped and I never drank again. I had no craving whatsoever."

But his medical problems were not over. Two years later, he had to go on dialysis. By 1994, he had suffered two serious episodes of high blood pressure. "I almost had a stroke and was taking Procardia— a high blood pressure medicine—when I went for more acupuncture treatments. It was amazing. After two or three visits, my pressure was normal and I had to stop the medicine. Now I go once every two weeks and my pressure has stayed normal for several months."

You may experience the same beneficial effects of acupuncture, but never stop taking high blood pressure or other medication without consulting both your Western and Chinese medicine doctors— and, if possible, having them talk with each other directly.

Phases, Worsley, or Van Nghi practitioners. Each approach has a tradition and a practice that has been refined and shaped so that it provides effective therapy. There is no right way.

As Charles Chace, a noted Chinese medicine scholar, points out in his article on the diversity of Chinese medicine, "While specific people throughout history may have believed they had a lock on the truth, the Chinese as a people never took this very seriously and never really strove toward a single truth. Chinese society as a whole never cared about a single truth, they just cared about what is useful, about what makes logical sense . . . a concept of absolute knowledge is not Chinese, and also the concept of either/or is not Chinese. Chinese medicine has historically allowed opposing points of view to exist simultaneously."[1]

TRADITIONAL CHINESE MEDICINE ACUPUNCTURE

Traditional Chinese Medicine (TCM) was consolidated after the Chinese revolution to unify diverse ancient practices into one coherent theoretical framework that would be especially useful for educating new practitioners. My practice is based on TCM, and predominantly I use the style of acupuncture that corresponds to that system of thought. It is based on the Eight Fundamental Patterns, Seven Emotions, Essential Substances, Organ Systems, and channels.

In TCM there are 365 basic acupuncture points located along twelve primary channels, eight extraordinary channels, and fifteen collaterals. Over the centuries, more than 2,500 points have been identified, but the average practitioner uses about 150.

JAPANESE ACUPUNCTURE

Japanese acupuncture focuses on clinical symptoms and is pragmatic. To Miki Shima, one of the leading proponents, Japanese acupuncture is a "healing art, based on the direct, nonconceptual and intuitive observations of the patient."

This system uses meridian (channel) therapy based on a diagnostic process that includes looking, listening, questioning, pulse diagnosis, palpation of meridians, and most importantly, abdominal diagnosis. Although there are several schools of abdominal diagnosis, they all focus on the belly as the area of the body where toxins become stagnant and therefore the source of illness. Organs and meridians are associated with sections of the abdomen and the texture, density, tenderness, appearance, and responses to touch of each section indicate specific disharmonies.

Other diagnostic techniques used by some Japanese acupuncturists include akabane and the O-ring test. Akabane is the practice of using a lit incense stick to test reaction to heat at the acu-points on the fingertips. The length of time it takes for a person to react to the heat indicates the nature of disharmony in the meridians. The O-ring test, designed by Dr. Y. Omura, a teacher of acupuncture, is a subtle system of testing muscle strength that is used in conjunction with herbal therapy and acupuncture.

When the practitioner uses acupuncture, he or she determines what acu-points to needle by palpation of the meridians. The Japanese school believes that the points are not found at fixed anatomical sites but move along the meridians, depending on the disharmony that's present.

In addition to their own system of acupuncture, Japanese practitioners use an herbal system called kampo, which is based on the original Chinese herbal text, the *Shang Han Lun*. Herbal formulas are prescribed based on symptoms without discussion of herbal properties. They rarely modify or add to formulas.

TRADITIONAL ACUPUNCTURE

Developed in England and the United States by J. R. Worsley, this school uses the Five Phases—metal, fire, water, earth, wood—and the channels associated with them for diagnosis and treatment. The main emphasis in traditional acupuncture is on the emotional and spiritual bases of disharmony.

Traditional acupuncture also emphasizes observation of facial color, interpretation of a person's vocal quality, and reading pulses using distinctly different pulse patterns than those used in TCM.

KOREAN ACUPUNCTURE

Korean or constitutional acupuncture is based on a system of identifying Qi imbalances through pulse diagnosis (modified from the Chinese) and determining which one of eight constitutional types a person falls into. Each constitutional type is linked with one organ system that is overactive and one that is depleted. For example, if your constitution is identified as *hespera,* that means you have a strong Lung and a weak Gallbladder.

Identification of constitutional type is then combined with the Five Phases understanding of the Organ Systems (wood is linked with Gallbladder and Liver Systems; fire with Heart and Small Intestine Systems; earth with Spleen and

Stomach Systems; metal with Lung and Large Intestine Systems; water with Kidney and Bladder Systems). This directs the practitioner to which of the Five Phases channel points to tonify or calm.

FUNCTIONS OF ACUPUNCTURE

Whatever type of acupuncture you receive, it will be effective for diagnosis, prevention, and treatment of disharmony.

DIAGNOSIS

When the body is in disharmony, acu-points along the channel become tender to the touch, alerting the practitioner to the location of disturbances in the channels and in associated Organ Systems. Some points become particularly tender when disease is present, and they offer vivid diagnostic help. For example, when the Lung or Heart System has disease, the Qi is detained in the crook of the elbow, making that area tender to the touch.

PREVENTION

Acupuncture maintains a balanced flow of Qi and Xue. By using it for regular tune-ups, you can keep your mind/body/spirit in harmony. Furthermore, acupuncture can be used to prevent disease from becoming more severe. You may have noticed that emotional and spiritual changes or disturbances often appear as the first sign of illness and imbalance. You don't quite feel right; you might have dream-disturbed sleep, or you might become easily irritated. These early clues to the onset of disease can be present in the body and can be identified through careful diagnosis before symptoms emerge. Acupuncture can then be used to re-balance the Qi and prevent the developing disharmony from turning into a full-blown illness or disorder.

TREATMENT

TCM acupuncture can adjust the flow of Essential Substances so that excesses are dispersed, deficiencies overcome, Dampness dispelled, Dryness eased, Cold warmed, and Heat cooled. It reestablishes balance and promotes a self-healing response by stimulating communication pathways within the body that promote tissue repair and natural pain control.

Used alone or in conjunction with herbal and dietary therapy and Qi Gong, acupuncture is a powerful force for promoting health and well-being.

> Alicia was suffering from chronic sciatica that had developed from an old sports injury. Painkillers only dulled her, physical therapy had not helped, and massage, although refreshing, had not offered lasting relief.
>
> She came to the clinic after she had been forced to postpone a much-needed vacation because she couldn't possibly sit on an airplane for five hours.
>
> Her treatment included acupuncture with electrostimulation, ear acupuncture, moxibustion and self-moxa, herbal therapy, and massage. After eight treatments, she had no more debilitating flare-ups and could sleep through the night. "You can stick a needle anywhere you like," she says with a laugh. "I don't question how, I just know this has given me my life back."

THE TAO OF ACUPUNCTURE

When a Chinese medicine practitioner uses acupuncture for diagnosis and treatment, he or she does not view the person's health as a phenomenon that is isolated from what is going on in the world outside or the general stages of life. Climate, geographic location, and age have an impact on the harmony of the mind/body/spirit and must be taken into consideration in evaluation or the development of a treatment plan.

CLIMATE

According to the ancient Chinese text, *Ling Shu,* "In spring, the pathogenic factors are most likely to attack the superficial layer; in summer, they are most likely to attack the skin; in autumn, they are most likely to attack the muscles; in winter, they are most likely to attack the bones and tendons." In treatment of such disorders, the *Ling Shu* also says that techniques should remain consistent with the seasons; "that's why in the spring and summer shallow acupuncture is generally used and in winter and autumn the deep acupuncture is preferred."

GEOGRAPHY

Geographic location has an impact on acupuncture treatment because climate affects diet and lifestyle, which in turn affects the way Essential Substances and Organ Systems function. People who live in desert areas, such as eastern Washington state or southern Arizona, or who live in cold, damp areas such as San

Francisco or London, need to have acupuncture treatments that are appropriate to such geographic conditions and help the mind/body/spirit maintain balance in the presence of such external influences.

INDIVIDUAL CONDITIONS

Acupuncture treatment is also tailored to the age, sex, and general constitution of the recipient. People of different ages and sexes have different physiologies. Sensitivity to acupuncture can vary widely. The *Ling Shu* explains these distinctions: "A middle-aged strong person with sufficient Qi and Xue and hard skin may, if being attacked by pathogenic factors, be treated by a deep needling with a needle retained for some time. . . . An infant has weak muscles and less volume of Qi and Xue, [so] acupuncture treatment is given twice a day with shallow needling and weak stimulation." The text also suggests deep needling for those engaged in physical labor and shallow needling for those who perform mental work.

HOW DOES ACUPUNCTURE WORK?

The science of how acupuncture works is of little concern to Traditional Chinese Medicine practitioners. Chinese medicine practitioners and the millions of surgical patients in China who have used acupuncture for an anesthesia care primarily about the effects of acupuncture.

There are six ways in which Traditional Chinese Medicine describes acupuncture's impact on the mind/body/spirit.

1. *Reinforcing* is used when there are no strong pathogenic forces at work in the body. It bolsters the Organ Systems and replenishes Yin, Yang, Qi, and Xue.
2. *Reducing* dispels pathogenic factors and breaks up stagnation. Reducing is never used in the presence of a Deficiency syndrome.
3. *Warming* removes blockages in the channels, nourishes Qi, dispels Cold, and restores Yang.
4. *Clearing* dispels Heat and remedies Heat syndromes with swift needling.
5. *Ascending* raises Qi, prevents sinking Qi, and prevents organ prolapse.
6. *Descending* sends Upward, Rebellious Qi downward and subdues Yang. It's never used when a Deficiency is present. (Note the difference between Sinking and Descending Qi: Sinking indicates what happens to Qi when it is not being supported or held up; descending indicates what happens to Qi when it is pushed down.)

Western science has two theories about the physiological effects of acupuncture when used as an anesthetic and as a remedy for disease.

The Gate Theory

This posits the idea that the nerves that transmit pain impulses from the body through the spinal cord to the brain have gates that can be opened or closed. There is debate about whether there are one, two, or four types of gates, since researchers are struggling to understand why needling the face can reduce the pain of abdominal surgery. Whatever the process of switching off pain, it appears that acupuncture may add an electronic message to neural pathways that causes the gate to open, interrupting the flow of information from the nerves such as pain. The pain impulses never make it to the brain.[2]

The Endorphin Theory

This theory, documented in animal and human trials, attributes acupuncture's pain-blocking effects to stimulation of the body's own painkillers, neurotransmitters called endorphins.[3] Other researchers have investigated the impact of stimulation of the endorphin system on the immune system. They suggest that acupuncture's curative powers may involve immunomodulation of prostaglandin hormones and interleukin-2.[4]

However, neither of these theories considers the interaction of acupuncture and Qi and Xue. Western science has not yet developed a quantitative measure for these Essential Substances.

ACUPUNCTURE TREATMENT

Acupuncture, whether done using traditional needles or by more modern techniques such as electrostimulation or laser, requires extensive training and should never be done on oneself. (You can, however, use acupressure and massage of acupoints, and there are complete instructions and explanations for you to follow in chapter 11.)

In the hands of a skilled practitioner, acupuncture is particularly effective for detoxification of drugs and alcohol; for pain control; for relief from depression, obsessive compulsive disorders, phobias, and anxiety attacks; for immunoregulation; to treat allergies, gynecological disorders, infertility, and digestive tract disturbances; to aid postoperative healing; and to ease the negative impact of Western cancer treatments.

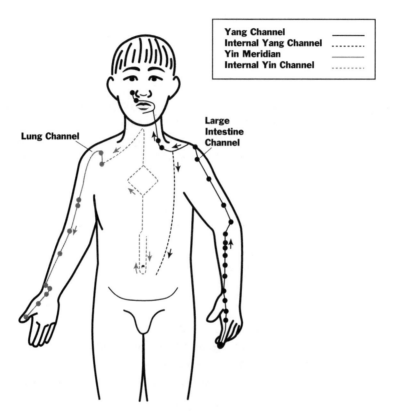

The Lung Channel of Hand-Taiyin
The Large Intestine Channel of Hand-Yangming

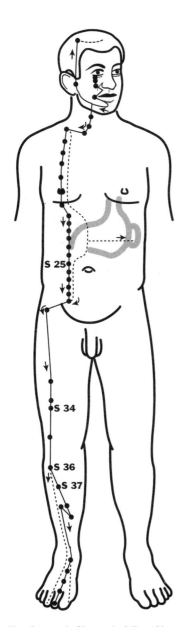

The Stomach Channel of Foot-Yangming

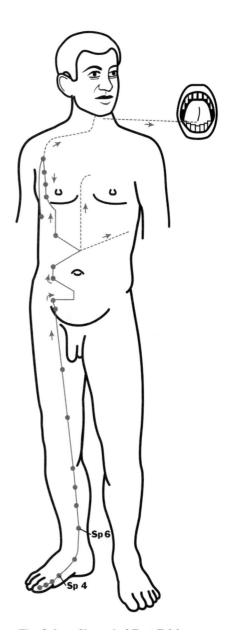

The Spleen Channel of Foot-Taiyin

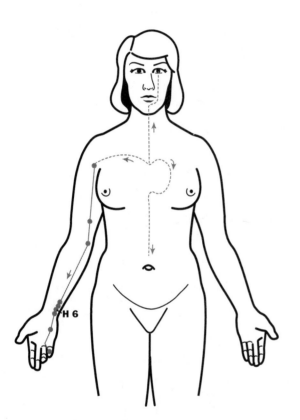

The Heart Channel of Hand-Shaoyin

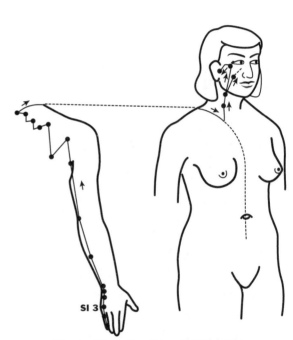

The Small Intestine Channel of Hand-Taiyang

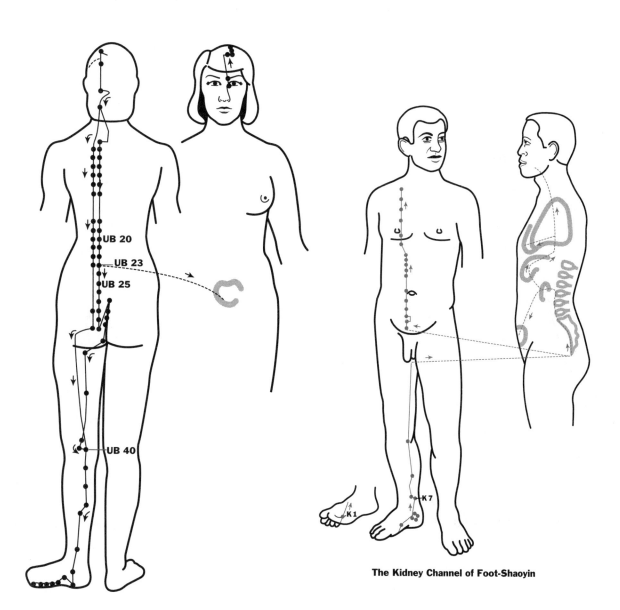

The Bladder Channel of Foot-Taiyang

The Kidney Channel of Foot-Shaoyin

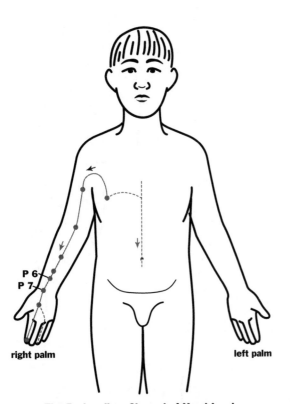

The Pericardium Channel of Hand-Jueyin

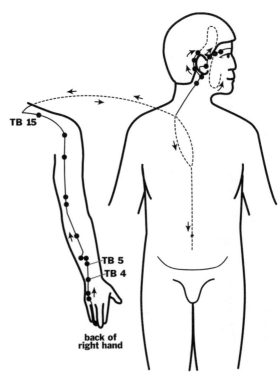

The Triple Burner (Sanjiao) Channel of Hand-Shaoyang

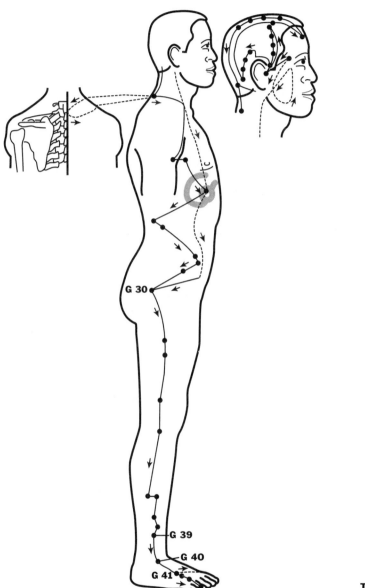

The Gallbladder Channel of Foot-Shaoyang

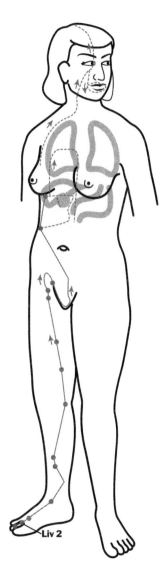

The Liver Channel of Foot-Jueyin

Charles, sixty-six, came to the clinic with severe shingles. He was taking massive doses of painkillers, hadn't slept through the night in months, and had taken a disability leave from work. He had already tried acupuncture with a Western physician to no avail, but we used electrostimulation in addition to a treatment called surrounding the dragon, which is designed specifically to remedy syndromes producing symptoms such as shingles.

"The needling feels good, like someone rocking you," he reported.

After the first treatment, he was pain free for six hours—the first relief he'd had in two months. After three treatments, he cut his use of painkillers dramatically and was able to sleep through the night. After one month of daily treatments, he was able to come every other day, then twice a week, and finally once a week. He went off painkillers completely.

Acupuncture and Clear Heat Chinese herbs, in conjunction with topical applications of vitamin E and white flower oil, reduced the skin and nerve irritation and pain.

"I'm considering going back to work now," says Charles.

EAR ACUPUNCTURE

Ear acupuncture, also known as auriculotherapy, has been practiced in China for hundreds of years. It is commonly used by Chinese medicine practitioners for diagnosis and treatment of Organ System disharmony. It works to control pain and is widely accepted by Western public health personnel as a highly effective system for helping people break and stay free of addictions to alcohol, hard drugs, and nicotine.

Self–ear acupressure is recommended for many disharmonies and can provide relief from a whole roster of acute problems such as headaches, nausea, anxiety, and digestive distress or menstrual discomfort. (For a diagram of the ear acu-points and information on self-massage, see chapter 11.)

COMMONLY ASKED QUESTIONS

Q: *Does acupuncture hurt?*

A: It shouldn't hurt to have the needles inserted, but there can be a slight pricking sensation when the needle first goes in. When there is a great deal of muscle tightness or Qi Stagnation, the sensation may be more intense.

   Once the needles are in place, the sensations range from none to a sharp tingle or a sense of wavy, pulsing turbulence. Again, there should never be any pain that feels wounding.

   On occasion, the sensation of Qi moving can seem overwhelming and some people request that a treatment be abbreviated, but even that is unusual. Most commonly, there is a sense of deep relaxation and a kind of floating quality.

Q: *How do you know where the points are?*

A: The acupuncturist can determine where to place the needles through a combination of several factors. Years of study and practice make the knowledge second nature. There are, however, identifiable anatomical landmarks for each point. Acupuncturists can also sense the points, which emanate a little beam of energy. For example, on the back of your hand at the crook between your thumb and first finger, about a half inch from the edge, is Large Intestine 4 (LI 4). If you take your index finger from your right hand and circle slowly about a quarter inch above the skin near the crook of your thumb, you will be able to feel the energy center for that point.

Q: *Is there blood?*

A: There is rarely any bleeding with acupuncture, although if someone has lots of small veins and capillaries close to the surface of the skin, it is more likely.

Q: *Is there any risk of disease transmission?*

A: There is no more risk of transmission of disease through acupuncture than there is through getting a flu shot. The use of sterile needles in a sanitary environment makes it a completely safe procedure. Whether your acupuncturist uses an autoclave to steam clean the needles or uses sterile disposable needles, you don't need to worry.

Q: *What are the risks?*

A: The risks are minor. According to a report from the U.S. Department of Health and Human Services, ". . . considering the number of patients treated [estimated nine to twelve million treatments a year] and the number of needles used per treatment [estimated average of six to eight], there are, however, remarkably few serious complications" (AAMA, 1981). There have been a handful of reported cases of infection transmission and there have been six reported cases of needles puncturing an organ. Broken needles are rare events. Other possible risks: acupuncture can induce labor in pregnant women, there can be an allergic reaction to the material in the acupuncture needles, and there are some people in China who are reportedly addicted to acupuncture, although it may be a sign of hypochondria.

MOXIBUSTION

Moxibustion uses burning herbs, placed on or near the body, to stimulate specific acupuncture points. This warms the channels and expels Cold and Dampness, creates a smooth flow of Qi and Xue, strengthens Yang Qi, prevents disease, and maintains health.

For hundreds of years, moxibustion has been partnered with acupuncture. According to the Chinese text *Introduction to Medicine*, "When a disease fails to respond to medication and acupuncture, moxibustion is suggested."

There are two basic forms of moxibustion: the cone and the stick. You can use both of them for self-care at home. You can buy the moxa herbs (often mugwort) at an herbalist.

The moxa cone is made by compressing the herb mixture, known as moxa wool, into a cone about the size of the upper part of your thumb. The cone is then burned on the body. One of the most common applications is to the navel, where it is effective in relieving abdominal pain, diarrhea, and easing excessive sweating, cold limbs, and a flagging pulse. When moxa cones are burned on other parts of the body, the effect is to ease disharmonies in channels and Organ Systems associated with those points.

USING THE MOXA CONE

At home, never place the moxa cone directly on your skin.

Make three cones. Place each one firmly on a slice of dry aconite about an eighth of an inch thick and set within arm's reach. Aconite is a special herb your practitioner can give you or you can buy from an herbalist. It may be toxic if ingested, but it is perfectly safe when used with the moxa cone. You may also use a slice of fresh ginger about an eighth of an inch thick that you have pierced with four or five small holes.

Lie down. Place a piece of clean cotton somewhere on your torso so you can retrieve it quickly if need be.

Put two tablespoons of salt in your navel and tamp down until smooth and flat. (If you have an "outtie," the Chinese texts suggest taking a long, wet noodle and forming a circle around the navel to contain the salt.)

Pick up the aconite with the cone on top. Light the cone—from the top if you want it to burn cooler and more slowly; from the bottom (don't light the aconite) if you want it to burn hotter and more rapidly. Place the aconite with the moxa on top of it over the salt.

If, as it burns, it becomes too hot, gently lift the moxa and aconite, slip the piece of cotton cloth over the salt, and set the aconite and moxa back in place. Note: Ginger tends to spread the heat more than aconite, and because it is damp, it doesn't offer as much insulation, so be especially careful not to burn your skin.

Let the moxa burn down. If it still feels too hot, remove the aconite and cotton and let the salt cool. Repeat three times. When you're done, save the aconite; brush off the salt.

To place moxa cones on other points, skip the salt and use a piece of cotton topped with a slice of ginger or aconite.

Moxa sticks, the size of a big cigar, are available prerolled from your practitioner or an herbalist. When lit, they are used like wands by circling their burning end over various acu-points. This method is particularly effective for treating painful joints and chronic problems such as dysmenorrhea, hernias, and abdominal pain.

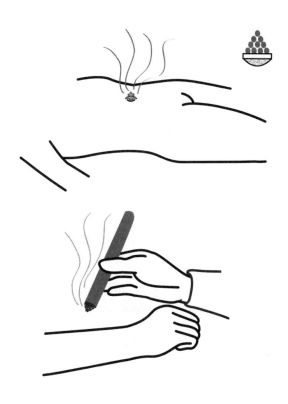

USING THE MOXA STICK

Mark the acu-points you want to heat with a small dot. Light the wand and let it burn until it begins to smoke. Holding it in the middle, bring the burning tip an inch from the skin. Move it slowly in a clockwise circle over the acu-point. If it feels too hot or the skin becomes too red, pull back in half-inch intervals until it feels warming but not burning. Repeat until the area feels bathed in warmth, you can sense the Qi flowing from that spot, and you feel relaxed.

TIP

To extinguish moxa cones or sticks, don't use water or try to smash out the fire. The best method is to cut off the supply of oxygen by wrapping the moxa in a piece of aluminum foil or placing it in a small container and sealing the top.

WHEN TO AVOID MOXIBUSTION

Moxa is contraindicated for heat and excess disharmonies or when there is a fever. Furthermore, pregnant women should avoid moxa on the abdominal and lumbosacral areas. Anyone with numbness in arms, legs, feet, or toes or who suffers from narcolepsy should not do moxa. No one should do moxa in bed.

WHERE TO APPLY MOXIBUSTION

- Ren 6—Located three fingers below the navel. Tonifies deficiency, tonifies Qi, strengthens the Kidney, and is good for gynecological disorders.
- Ren 8—Located in the navel. Tonifies Yang, warms the abdomen, strengthens Qi, and is good for all types of diarrhea and coldness.
- Stomach 36—Located four fingers below the knee, near the bone on the outer side of the leg. This is a major Qi point on the body and tonifies and regulates Qi, harmonizes the Stomach and the Spleen, and is good for digestive disorders and lack of energy.
- Spleen 6—Four fingers above the bone that sticks out of the inner ankle. Known as the Three Yin meeting point, it tonifies the Spleen, Kidney, and Liver and is good for gynecologic and digestive disorders.
- Ren 12—Halfway between the navel and the tip of the sternum. Effective in dispelling Dampness and treating digestive problems associated with Cold.

WORLD HEALTH ORGANIZATION'S RECOGNIZED APPLICATIONS FOR ACUPUNCTURE

The World Health Organization (WHO) released a list of diseases that it feels lend themselves to acupuncture treatment either for pain control or medical therapy. Interestingly, although the United States is a member of WHO, many United States insurance companies are reluctant to recognize acupuncture as a valid medical treatment.

Upper respiratory tract

Acute sinusitis

Acute rhinitis

Common cold

Acute tonsillitis

Respiratory System

Acute bronchitis

Bronchial asthma (most effective in children and patients without complicating diseases)

Disorders of the eye

Acute conjunctivitis

Central retinitis

Myopia in children

Cataract without complications

Disorders of the mouth

Toothache

Postextraction pain

Gingivitis

Acute and chronic pharyngitis

Gastrointestinal disorders

Spasm of the esophagus and cardia

Hiccup

Gastroptosis

Acute and chronic gastritis

Gastric hyperacidity

Chronic duodenal ulcer (pain relief)

Acute duodenal ulcer (without complications)

Acute and chronic colitis

Acute bacterial dysentery

Constipation

Diarrhea

Paralytic ileus

Neurological and musculoskeletal disorders

Headache

Migraine

Trigeminal neuralgia

Facial palsy (early stage, i.e., three to six months)

Pareses following stroke

Sequelae of poliomyelitis (within 6 months)

Meniere's disease

Nocturnal enuresis

Intercostal neuralgia

Cervicobrachial syndrome

Frozen shoulder

Tennis elbow

Sciatica

Low back pain

Osteoarthritis

CHAPTER TEN

Qi Gong

Chinese Exercise and Meditation

Wholeness = Dietary Guidelines + Herbs + Acupuncture + **Qi Gong**

Exercise/meditation is the fourth pillar of Chinese medicine therapy. Without its Qi-balancing effects and benefits to mind/body/spirit, wholeness cannot be achieved.

I recommend Qi Gong to many of my clients as part of a total program. Although I am not an expert in the practice of Qi Gong, I do know how important it is to the process of restoring harmony. For those who are not particularly interested in exercising, it offers immediate gratification—you feel good right away—without having to go through a painful aerobics routine, joining some overcrowded health club, or spending money on equipment. For those who are exercise enthusiasts, it offers the health benefits of running or weight training without the risks. And it does what other forms of exercise cannot do: it strengthens and harmonizes the flow of Qi.

So many people come into the clinic suffering from the fanatic pursuit of Western exercise: sore muscles, bruised bones, twisted ankles, sore backs, tension and stress. These frequent injuries occur in part because the concept of exercise has become distorted. Feel the burn. Bop till you drop. No pain, no gain. We battle to make our bodies look like the modern ideal, which has little or nothing to do with genuine healthfulness. We compete with one another for glory, prestige and ego gratification. This notion of exercise often injures the mind/body/spirit; it makes us sore and exhausted instead of agile and refreshed. Too often, for some people, it damages the Qi by reducing energy. They end up feeling generally fatigued and lousy. For other people, exercise has become a kind of poison to the system instead of an expression of the joyous unity of mind/body/spirit.

In contrast, Qi Gong exercise/meditation is a unified process dedicated to creating balance, strength, agility, and grace that assures vitality through old age. Qi Gong and its offshoots, Kung Fu and Tai Chi, have evolved as the logical outcome of the Tao and the recognition that the body is infused with Qi, which must be nurtured and tended to if wholeness is to prevail.

Historically, many different groups have used Qi Gong. The pragmatic followers of Confucius found its manipulation of Qi an aid in managing the demands of the world at large. Taoists thought of Qi Gong as a way to empower their pursuit of immortality and self-improvement. Buddhist monks, relying heavily on meditative/breathing techniques, used Qi Gong to help them escape the confines of earthly woes and to increase strength. A monk developed the first text of muscle-training routines in the sixth century, when he became alarmed by the physical weakness of his fellow monks. His *Yi Gin Ching* (Muscle Development Classic) laid out ways to use concentration to develop Qi and increase circulated Qi—and Kung Fu was born.

Eventually, the concept of working with Qi to increase mental, spiritual, and physical powers was embraced by many Chinese schools of thought and practice. Today, millions of people practice various forms of Qi Gong.

Following is an introduction to several of the basic techniques. We hope that you will integrate them into your exercise routines, expanding your definition of physical fitness and experimenting with ways of combining Eastern exercise with Western sports activities. Your guide is Larry Wong, an accomplished practitioner and teacher.

QI GONG 101: UNDERSTANDING THE CHINESE CONCEPT OF EXERCISE/MEDITATION BY LARRY WONG

Welcome. I am going to introduce you to what I know of the arts of Qi Gong. I urge you to keep in mind that there are many approaches to Qi Gong. Each one provides far-reaching health benefits. I will share only a few of those with you, but that doesn't mean that one method is inherently better than another. With Qi Gong, you may learn the principles and gain the benefits from any number of approaches.

WHAT IS QI GONG?

Qi Gong, which combines meditative and physically active elements, is the basic exercise system within Chinese medicine. Qi Gong practice is designed to help you preserve your Jing, strengthen and balance the flow of Qi, and enlighten your Shen. Its dynamic exercises and meditations have Yin and Yang aspects: the Yin is being it; the Yang is doing it. Yin exercises are expressed through relaxed stretching, visualization, and breathing; Yang exercises are expressed in a more aerobic or dynamic way. They are particularly effective for immune stimulation. In China, Qi Gong is used extensively for people with cancer.

Qi Gong's physical and spiritual routines move Qi energy through the twelve main channels and eight extra channels, balancing that energy, smoothing the flow, and strengthening it. Chinese medicine uses Qi Gong to maintain health, prevent illness, and extend longevity because it is a powerful tool for maintaining and restoring harmony to the Organ Systems, Essential Substances, and channels. Qi Gong is also used for nonmedical purposes: for fighting and for pursuing enlightenment.

Anyone of any age or physical condition can do Qi Gong. You don't have to be able to run a marathon or bench press a car to pursue healthfulness and enjoy the benefits. When you design your exercise/meditation practice, you will pick what suits your individual constitution. Some of us are born with one type of constitution, some with another. We each have inherited imbalances that we cannot control but with which we must work. That's why for some people it is easier to achieve balance and strength than for others. Whatever your nature, Qi Gong can help you become the most balanced you can be.

Qi Gong is truly a system for a lifetime. That's why so many people over sixty in China practice Qi Gong and Tai Chi. The effects may be powerful, but the routines themselves are usually gentle. Even the dynamic exercises—some of which explode the Qi—use forcefulness in different ways than in the West.

MAINTAINING HEALTH

Qi Gong helps maintain health by creating a state of mental and physical calmness, which indicates that Qi is balanced and harmonious. This allows the mind/body/spirit to function most efficiently, with the least amount of stress.

When you start practicing Qi Gong, the primary goal is to concentrate on letting go, letting go, letting go. That's because most imbalance comes from holding on to too much for too long. Most of us are familiar with the physical strength of muscles, and when we think about exercising, we think in terms of tensing muscles. Qi is different. Qi strength is revealed by a smooth, calm, concentrated effort that is free of stress and does not pit one part of the body against another.

MANAGING ILLNESS

It's harder to remedy an illness than to prevent it, and Qi Gong has powerful preventive effects. However, when disharmony becomes apparent, Qi Gong also can play a crucial role in restoring harmony.

Qi Gong movement and postures are shaped by the principle of Yin/Yang: the complementary interrelationship of qualities such as fast and slow, hard and soft, excess and deficiency, external and internal. Qi Gong uses these contrasting and complementary qualities to restore harmony to the Essential Substances, Organ Systems and channels.

EXTENDING LONGEVITY

In China, the use of Qi Gong for maintaining health and curing illness did not satisfy those Buddhists and Taoists who engaged in more rigorous self-discipline. They wanted to be able to amplify the power of Qi and make the internal Organ Systems even stronger. This arcane use of Qi Gong was confined mostly to monasteries and the techniques have not been much publicized. One of the most difficult and profoundly effective techniques is called Marrow Washing Qi Gong. Practitioners learn to master the intricate manipulation of Qi, infusing the eight extraordinary channels with Qi, and then guiding the Qi through the channels to the bone marrow to cleanse and energize it. The result, according to religious tradition, is that monks can extend their life span to 150 years or more. The Taoists have a saying: "One hundred and twenty years means dying young."

Although few if any of us can devote our lives to the stern practices of the monks, the health benefits of Qi Gong certainly do improve the quality of life of everyone who practices it.

WAGING COMBAT

Around 500 A.D. in the Liang Dynasty, Qi Gong was adopted by various martial arts to increase stamina and power. For the most part, the breathing, concentration, and agility were assets to the warriors and improved their well-being.

ATTAINING ENLIGHTENMENT

Buddhist monks who use Qi Gong in their pursuit of higher consciousness and enlightenment concentrate on Qi Gong's ability to influence their Shen. Mastering Marrow Washing allows the practitioner to gain so much control over the flow of Qi that he or she can direct it into the forehead and elevate consciousness. The rest of us do enjoy the influence of Qi Gong on our Shen but at a lower level.

Whatever reason you do Qi Gong, the practice should raise your Qi to a higher state if you increase concentration, practice controlled breathing, and execute the Qi Gong routines.

THE BASIC TECHNIQUES

Concentration

Concentration leads to and results from Qi awareness, breathing techniques, and Qi Gong exercises. It is a process of focusing in and letting go at the same time. Focusing does not mean that you wrinkle up your forehead and strain to pay attention. Instead, through deep relaxation and expanding your consciousness you are able to create a frame of mind that is large enough to encompass your entire body/mind/spirit's functions, yet focused enough to allow outside distractions, worries, and everyday hassles to drift away.

This inward focus that expands outward to join you with the rhythms of the universe epitomizes Yin/Yang. Yin tends to be more expansive and Yang more concentrated. You discover your Yin/Yang balance by treating Yin and Yang as ingredients in a recipe: add a bit more Yin, a dash of Yang to make the mixture suit your constitution or circumstances. Some people need more or less Yin or Yang in various situations. Extending the Qi exercise on page 161 provides a clear demonstration of how you can practice establishing your balanced blend of Yin and Yang.

You will find that as you do exercise/meditation, you become more adept at this form of concentration, since it is the natural expression of the practice. As you learn to concentrate more effectively, you will find you have greater power to affect Qi through the various Qi Gong exercises in this chapter or through the use of other focused meditations and Tai Chi.

Breathing

Lao Tzu, from the sixth century B.C., first described breathing techniques as a way to stimulate Qi. From there, two types of breathing evolved: Buddha's Breath and Taoist's Breath. Both methods infuse the body with Qi and help focus meditation.

Buddha's Breath   When you inhale, extend your abdomen, filling it with air. When you exhale, contract your abdomen, expelling the air from the bottom of your lungs first and then pushing it up and out until your abdomen and chest are deflated. You may want to practice inhaling for a slow count of eight and exhaling for a count of sixteen. As you breathe in and out, imagine inviting your Qi to flow through the channels. Use your mind to invite the Qi to flow; you want to guide the flow, not tug at it or push it.

Taoist's Breath   The pattern is the opposite of above. When you breathe in, you contract your abdominal muscles. When you exhale you relax the torso and lungs.

Qi Gong Routines

There are two basic types of Qi Gong activities: Wei Dan (external elixir) and Nei Dan (internal elixir). Both focus on strengthening and balancing the Qi by using dynamic routines and still postures, but they approach the tasks in two different ways.

Wei Dan   This practice focuses on the muscles in order to build up Qi until it becomes so concentrated that it overflows and runs out from where it has collected, through the channels, and into all parts of the body.

In dynamic, moving Wei Dan exercises, muscles are tensed and released over and over again with complete concentration. **The tension should be as light as possible, since tension causes Qi Stagnation—the very antithesis of what you want to accomplish. In fact, it is often suggested that you simply *imagine* that you are tensing the muscles.** After several minutes, the generated Qi warms the muscles.

Typical routines that use dynamic, moving Wei Dan exercises include the Dan Mo or Muscle/Tendon Changing Classic. In this, you slightly tense or imagine you are tensing isolated limb muscles such as the forearm, the palm, the wrist, the biceps, the shoulder, and then relax completely. Concentration and breath control are vital components of the process.

There are other moving Wei Dan routines that call for moving legs, torso, and arms into specific positions to relax or massage the Organ Systems. For example, you may extend and stretch your arms over your head, hold, and relax, thus massaging the Lung channel and Lung Organ System more enthusiastically than with the less mobile Dan Mo style.

In the still Wei Dan exercises, muscle groups are targeted but not tensed. For example, hold your arms fully extended, palms down, out to the side of your body. Don't tighten muscles, but hold that position for at least a minute—building up to longer—until the arms begin to shake or feel warm. When you let your arms fall to your sides and relax, shrugging your shoulder muscles and shaking your hands gently, the accumulated Qi is sent coursing out through the channels. In this manner, Qi is stimulated at various locations in the body by continual muscular exertion combined with concentration.

Wei Dan practice is relatively simple to learn and provides immediate benefits, but it is not a lesser form of Qi Gong. Even masters of the more arcane processes use Wei Dan for its Qi strengthening powers.

Qi can also be stimulated to a higher state through acupuncture, acupressure, and massage, which are considered Wei Dan exercises.

Nei Dan   This is a more demanding, less easy to master, and more time-consuming form of Qi Gong. It uses mental powers to direct Qi through the channels. You must have a teacher to guide you and to help you avoid the potential risks associated with doing the practice incorrectly.

In one Nei Dan exercise, you concentrate Qi in a spot an inch and a half below the navel (the dan-tien) and then disperse it through the body using the powers of the mind. Qi may travel three pathways:

1. *The Fire Path:* In the Fire Path, you build Qi in the abdomen through breathing and/or thought, and once it accumulates sufficiently, you direct it with your mind along the two extra channels known as the conception channel and the governing channel. This is known as the Small Circulation.

The next level is to move Qi through the remaining six extra channels. This is called the Grand Circulation.

2. *The Wind Path:* On this path, Qi moves in the opposite direction from that of the Fire Path. See illustration.

3. *The Water Path:* This is the path through the spine and is used in Marrow Washing to prolong life and increase enlightenment.

THE QI GONG CLASS

This is a beginning class, designed to help you become sensitive to the positive benefits of Qi Gong and to prepare you for taking classes with a teacher who can guide you through the learning process. One word about teachers: make sure you find one who has a watchful eye, is compassionate, can perceive your individual blocks, and who can direct you to exercises and routines that release those blocks. Not all great masters make good teachers, for a teacher must be able not only to do the Qi Gong well but to communicate effectively.

The first part of the class is devoted to improving your awareness of tension and blocks in your body so you can shed unnecessary stress. If you practice Qi Gong without letting go of blocks and tension, it will impair your practice and your Qi will not flow evenly or as well as it can.

The next step is to begin to be aware of your internal organs and to tune in to the flow of Qi throughout the body. Then you're ready to explore breathing exercises and basic Qi Gong routines.

As you travel through these steps, please remember that Qi Gong is a process of building awareness, and however you are comfortable doing the routines is what's right for you at that time.

LOOSENING UP EXERCISES (10–15 MINUTES)

Exercise One: Gentle Sway

For five minutes, move both whole arms from the shoulders in a gentle swinging motion. The motion itself is initiated from the waist. Twist from the waist as though your torso were a washcloth that you were wringing out. Don't twist from the knees or you may harm them. Furthermore, twisting from the waist provides a massage to the internal organs and provides the full benefits of the exercise.

To get started, move your arms side to side across your torso, then back to front. Keep your knees slightly bent. Let your hips sway. Allow the mind to clear. Focus, at first, on the release of unnecessary and unconscious stress. After several weeks, you may shift your focus so that you think only about the swaying of your arms and the motion of Qi.

This introduces the concept of being mindful of the present, much the same concept as found in Zen walking.

Exercise Two: The Bounce

In the beginning, try this for one to three minutes.

With feet parallel and about shoulder's width apart, bounce with knees loose and arms hanging at the sides like a wet noodle—they feel empty and neutral. This is the zero position for arms. When you are bouncing back and forth, your arms in zero should get a nice jiggling effect.

Keep shoulders natural; neither pull them back or let them slump forward too much.

When the zero position is used on the whole body, you should receive a feeling of deep relaxation and your internal organs and skin should hang down. This process brings awareness of internal tension so that you can do something to dispel it, if you choose.

The combination of exercises one and two gently massages and tonifies the Organ Systems, which helps promote longevity.

QI AWARENESS EXERCISES

Exercise One: Accordion

In this exercise, you feel the Qi by using your hands like the bellows of an accordion or a bicycle pump.

Close your eyes halfway. Clear your mind and concentrate your attention on your palms.

Allow your breath to become slow, easy, without force. In a way, you are creating the very lightest trance.

Bring your hands together, palms touching and fingers pointing upward. The palm chakras, called Laogong, located in the center of the palm, should be touching. These chakras are areas where Qi can be felt emanating from the body.

Slowly move your hands, keeping the chakras aligned. When they are about twelve inches apart, slowly move them together, using the least amount of physical effort possible. You will be compressing the air between them like an accordion would.

Feel a warm or tingling sensation at the chakra points on your palms.

Move your hands slowly back and forth, varying the range of the bellows.

Repeat the accordion technique in different directions: horizontally, vertically, and diagonally.

This exercise cultivates Qi, builds awareness, and sensitizes your self. When you feel Qi for the first time, it changes your mind-set.

VARIATION OUT

Exercise Two: Making the Point

Your index finger is a powerful way of directing Qi. If you are right-handed, use your right index finger; if left-handed, use your left index finger. Point it directly at the flat palm of your other hand. That hand should be perpendicular to the floor with your fingers pointing straight up.

Use your index finger like a paint brush to swab back and forth across your palm. Begin with your fingertip about eight inches from your palm. Slowly move it closer and farther away, swabbing all the time.

You may feel a tickling sensation, a cooling, or a warming of your palm.

Exercise Three: Extending the Qi

Those with Qi Deficiencies should perform this exercise with their eyes half closed in order to cultivate and accumulate Qi.

If you have Stagnant Qi, the exercise may be done with the eyes fully open when you inhale swiftly through your nostrils and open or half closed when you exhale.

You should exercise caution about practicing Qi exercises at home—without a teacher nearby—because they are powerful and Qi can leak out your eyes.

Once you can sense the Qi, exercise your intention (which is the mind/spirit part of the exercise) and use your mind to move your Qi out from your body, expanding the zone in which you are comfortable. You may allow the Qi to drift out on the exhalation and then hold it there as you inhale.

First, move the Qi into an orbit one inch from your skin. In increments of six inches, move it outward, aiming for three feet, but find the point where you are comfortable with it. Then bring it back in until it returns close to your body.

This exercise allows you to communicate with your Qi. By increasing the distance away from your body that you can feel Qi, you expand your area of comfort—your field of generosity—in the world around you. You will have less fear and greater abilities. By being able to bring your Qi halo in to skin level (or inside your skin) you may become more centered, calm, more self-assured. When you have learned to be comfortable expanding **and** contracting your Qi, you will feel stronger, healthier, and more in harmony internally and externally.

Exercise Four: Pumping the Qi

This is a tricky exercise that moves the Qi along the two connecting extraordinary channels, the Du Mai and Ren Mai. You may think of it as *evolve, devolve,* since your posture goes from a slumped, gorilla-like stance to an upright, extended pose. It is adapted from the Wild Goose routine.

The first position pushes the Qi down. As your hands push flat down, your spine and head straighten upward. Then, as you allow the Qi to flow back upward, your hands rise, elbows bent and palms parallel to the floor. Your shoulders hunch. Repeat six or seven times, inhaling as hands come up and exhaling as hands go down.

When you are comfortable with the previous exercise, you may combine it with a slow, intentional walk forward: left knee bent and raised in exaggerated stepping motion. When your knee comes up, your hands go down and back, and your spine straightens; when your foot touches the ground, your hands come up, and your back hunches. Place your feet very gently on the ground and allow each step to proceed in slow motion, at a tempo that soothes and relaxes. Remember to maintain your breathing pattern, too. Inhale as your hands come up and your shoulders hunch. Exhale slowly, expanding your chest as you straighten your back. If this feels awkward, don't despair; even in a classroom situation, it takes a while to catch on to what to do.

Exercise Five: Blending Qi

This exercise should help you become aware of various resonations of Qi and help you learn to blend them into a harmonious flow.

Stand with your feet a shoulder's width apart, knees slightly bent. Allow your hands and arms to hang at your sides.

Shift your weight slightly to the balls of your feet. Simply be aware of the front side of your body. Concentrate on the channels that pass along the front of your legs and torso, the top of your hands and arms, your face.

After one minute, shift your weight to your heels. Become aware of the back of your body: the back of your head, your arms, your spine, your legs. With practice, you may hold these postures for up to five minutes or longer.

You can also do this for the left and right sides of the body.

In each instance, you may want to become aware of each section of your body. For example, the side of the head, the side of the arm and torso, the outer hip, the side of the leg and ankle, the length of the foot. This make the exercise a meditation.

Now, shifting to a more Nei Dan form of Qi Gong, repeat the first three steps, but the motion should not be detectable visually. Use your mind to shift your weight forward and backward, feeling your Qi flowing along the front and back of your body.

Next, try to feel your Qi flowing along your back and front simultaneously.

Students are often bewildered by the idea of feeling two sensations at the same time, but a useful analogy is to think of the color yellow and the color blue. When you blend those two colors, you produce green. That green then becomes its own entity with its own wavelength. The same is true of blending the Qi from your front and from your back; the blend becomes another entity with its own resonation.

BREATHING EXERCISES

Breathing can direct Qi through the body like the wind filling the sails of a ship. Breathing exercises can invigorate or sedate, depending on how you use them.

On alternate days, practice this routine using Buddha's and Taoist's breathing techniques.

Sit on the floor with legs crossed in lotus or cross-legged style. This is important so that Qi does not enter and become stagnated in the lower body, but follows the breathing path through the torso and the head.

Inhale to a count of four to eight, depending on what you are comfortable with. For Buddha's breath, extend your belly, filling it up from the bottom. For Taoist's breath, inhale, contracting your abdomen; exhale letting your abdomen relax outward.

As you inhale, turn your attention to your nose. Guide the Qi downward from your nose toward a spot in your abdomen about one to two inches below the navel. This is the dan-tien, and women should not concentrate on it during their periods. Concentrate on the solar plexus, instead.

Exhale to a count of eight to sixteen and move the Qi down the torso around the pelvic region and up to the tailbone.

Inhale and move the Qi up the back to the top of the shoulders.

Exhale and move the Qi up the back of the head and back to the nose.

If you cannot feel the Qi clearly, patience and practice will make it more apparent. Then, once you are comfortable with this practice, you may increase the pace by completing the cycle in one inhalation and one exhalation. On inhalation, move Qi from the nose to the tailbone. On exhalation, move Qi from the tailbone back to the nose.

MEDITATION

The following meditations are those used at Chicken Soup Chinese Medicine clinic.

As a beginner, you want to allow yourself the time and pleasure of learning to meditate. If it feels awkward or you have difficulty maintaining concentration, take a step back.

Don't set your standards too high. If you expect too much too soon, you disturb your mind/body/spirit and promote restlessness, frustration and stress. This may defeat the whole purpose of meditation.

Your first goal should be simply to be quiet, relaxed and comfortable for a few minutes.

Try to meditate in a comfortable environment. As you progress, distractions will become less of a problem, but in the beginning, you want to eliminate as many distractions as possible. Choose a quiet room that is not so warm that you fall asleep or so cold that you tense up. Wear only loose-fitting clothing. Use meditation music to help block outside noise if need be.

Find a posture that works for you. Not everyone can sit on the floor in a full or half lotus or cross-legged. You may want to lie down, sit in a straight-backed chair, or stand.

Don't eat heavy foods or drink alcohol or caffeine before meditating.

Don't hold on to disturbing thoughts. One of the goals of meditation is to disconnect from worries. If you've had a tough day at work or a disagreement with your spouse or are worried about money, each exhalation of breath is a chance to let a piece of that tension dissipate.

Qi Meditation

The following is a meditation/visualization that is designed to help you tune into the motion of Qi throughout the channels and to help in the body's natural process of self-healing.

The first few times you do this meditation, have someone read it to you in a gentle, slow voice, cuing you as to the steps. You can also tape this in your own voice and listen to it as you go through the meditation. Eventually, you will be able to go through the steps silently.

Sit comfortably in a chair or lie down on your back on a mat.

Allow your body to begin to relax. Close your eyes. Close your mouth and place the tip of your tongue against the roof of your mouth—this connects the Yin and Yang channels and allows for Qi flow.

With your eyes closed, bring your attention to the area around and below your navel; in Japanese it is called the *hara;* in Chinese, the *dan-tien.* This is one area where Qi is stored.

Allow yourself to begin to breathe into the area. You may use either breathing technique.

As you breathe into the abdomen, into the belly, into the dan-tien, notice a warmth from the center of the abdomen, which begins as a small glow and gets brighter and brighter until there is a ball of light filling your abdomen. Allow yourself to feel this ball of light, any color that you'd like.

As you breathe, notice the energy moving up into the area of your Heart and opening up into your chest.

Now feel it move to the area in front of the arm, just below the shoulder bone. This energy moves from the area below the shoulder bone, down the outside of the arm, all the way to the thumb, on the inside of the thumb. Feel the warmth and the movement of energy down the Lung channel.

When it gets to the end of the channel at the tip of the thumb, move your focus over to the index finger, where the Large Intestine channel begins.

The Qi then moves through the hand, up the outside of the arm, coming up over the shoulder, up the side of the neck, and up to the outside of the nose.

Then it moves to the Stomach channel, which begins below the eye. It flows down the neck, over the front of the body, through the chest, down outside the navel, around the pubic area, then down the outside of the leg, to a very important point, just below the knee, where the energy of the body becomes very strong. It then moves on down across the front of the foot and into the top of the toes, where it meets the Spleen channel.

The Spleen channel allows food energy to move through the body and impacts digestion.

Begin inside the big toe, coming up the arch of the foot, in front of the ankle bone, on the inside of the leg, all the way up by the knee, continuing inside the leg, and up the front of the body, curving around the ribs, and ending in the costal area. The Spleen channel then connects internally with the Heart.

The Heart channel emerges from the heart into the center of the armpit, moving down the inside of the arm, all the way to the small finger, where it attaches to the Small Intestine channel.

The Small Intestine channel is a very good channel to help open up the brain. This channel runs up the outside of the arm, coming all the way back up, across the scapula, up the back of the neck and around the ear, where it ends in front of the ear.

This connects to the Bladder channel, the longest channel, at the inside of the eye.

From the eye, the channel comes up across the top of the head, down the back of the neck, where it splits into two parallel lines that extend down the whole back on either side of the spine, connecting the organs together.

The two rows of the Bladder channel that are side by side then connect again at the back of the buttocks, coming down the back of the middle of the leg, through the knee, all the way down the leg, around the ankle bones, and into the little toe.

The Bladder channel connects with the Kidney channel on the very bottom of the foot. The Kidney channel moves up from the foot, around the inside of the ankle, all the way up the inside of the leg, up around the navel. This channel comes all the way up to the upper part of the chest, where there are some of the most important points in Chinese medicine for meditation and connection with the Shen.

Here the Kidney channel connects with the Pericardium channel, which starts in front of the arm, moves down the very middle of the arm into the palm of the hand, to the middle finger, where it then connects with the Triple Burner channel, the channel that helps to regulate the temperature of our bodies. This begins on the fourth finger, comes up over the top of the hand, all the way up the arm and around the elbow, over the shoulder, coming up the neck and around the ear, where it connects with the Gallbladder channel.

The Gallbladder channel is the most crooked channel on the body. It zigzags across the top of the head, comes down the back of the neck, across the shoulder, down the side of the body, zigzagging again on the side of the body, all the way down over the hip and the deepest point in the muscle of the body in the buttocks, then moving down the side of the leg, all the way down to the top of the toes, to the fourth toe.

You pick up the Liver channel on the big toe. It comes across the top of the foot, and again toward the inside of the foot and around the ankle, up the middle of the inside of the leg by the knee, all the way up the inside of the leg. This channel circles the genital area, coming up into the rib cage near the Liver, yet on both sides of the body. Then we return again to the Lungs.

Once you have completed the cycle, sit or lie peacefully, allowing yourself time to make the transition back to your surrounding environment in a graceful manner.

Lotus Blossom Meditation

This is a brief meditation that can be done almost anywhere, anytime you feel the need to ease stress or allow your feelings of affection and connection to expand.

Sit peacefully, breathing evenly.

Half close your eyes.

Inhale slowly, filling your body with air.

At the same time, concentrate your attention on your fourth chakra, which is located at your breastbone in the center of your chest.

Imagine a beautiful lotus blossom. Its petals are closed and its scent but a promise.

As you exhale, see that blossom unfold. The velvety, smooth petals extend, reaching out, releasing a beautiful scent.

Inhale and smell the fragrant aroma.

The petals are opening ever farther. And as they open, you feel your heart and chest opening up to the world, expanding, relaxing.

You may extend the opening petals as far as you want. Feel your heart open in the same proportion.

When you have arrived at an openness that is comfortable, hold it there as you enjoy the scent of the flower and breathe in and out slowly.

You may practice this meditation concentrating on a chakra, or energy center: particularly effective are the third chakra, located at the diaphragm, and the second chakra, located below the navel in the dan-tien or hara area.

CHAPTER ELEVEN

The Healing Touch

Qi Gong Massage and Other Forms of Body Therapy

Massage, whether done solo, with a partner, or by a professional massage therapist, offers the energy of acupuncture, the serenity of meditation and the spiritual refreshment that comes through being touched. Massage is an important part of your everyday health care routine. Just as you strive to integrate the dietary guidelines from chapter 8 and the exercise/meditation guidelines from chapter 10 into your daily self-care habits, so should you make room for massage as part of the routine you follow to strengthen your immune system and maintain your balance.

In this chapter we look at Chinese Qi Gong self-massage, self-acupressure, self-ear acupressure, Shiatsu for partners, and Western reflexology for the foot and hand to do with a partner or by yourself. There are many other forms of massage, each valuable for restoring harmony. Although they are not presented in detail in this book, you may want to explore them. They can be integrated into your comprehensive program for preventive care or to treat disharmony. In addition to massage, the chapter also offers soaks, saunas, and compresses to be used for deep muscle relaxation, stress reduction, and pain relief in conjunction with massage or by themselves.

QI GONG MASSAGE

Qi Gong massage is an extension of Qi Gong exercise/meditation. Among the more skilled masters of the art, self-massage can be done with the mind, moving Qi and Xue through the channels, relaxing muscles, and massaging Organ Systems mentally. For the rest of us, manual Qi Gong massage—done on ourselves or with a partner or practitioner—is an important part of any preventive health care program, since regular massage helps nourish the mind/body/spirit and maintains harmony in all systems.

If you exercise three or more times a week, go through the complete ten-step self-massage once a week. Use the specific self-massage routines for hand, ear, head, or foot as you feel the need.

If you are sedentary, have an injury that's preventing you from exercising, or you simply find you're stuck at the desk and cannot exercise for a given period of time, do the foot and head massage every other day; complete the ten-step self-massage program once or twice a week. You will help prevent the formation of disharmonies in the flow of Essential Substances and consequent problems in the Organ Systems.

The benefits of Qi Gong massage include tonification of the channels to improve circulation of Essential Substances, particularly Qi and Xue; dilation of the blood vessels; stimulation of the lymph system and elimination of wastes and toxins; improved muscle tone; relief of stress and promotion of relaxation and sleep; and it just makes you feel good.

WARNING

You should not perform self-massage or have a massage done to you on any area where you have a skin eruption, a localized infection, swelling, localized malignancies, or where you've had recent surgery.

Pregnant women should have massage on the abdomen and torso from a professional massage therapist only.

TEN-STEP QI-XUE SELF-MASSAGE

Based on the flow of the Essential Substances through the channels and Organ Systems, this massage series provides you with a complete relaxation and rejuvenation routine. You may use all or any part of it any time you feel the need of a little repair work and a bit of TLC.[1]

Establish a slow, rhythmic pattern of breathing while doing self-massage. Inhale slowly for the count of three and exhale slowly for the count of six. As you become more comfortable with this entire series of exercises, try to inhale every time you change the position of your hands and exhale while you massage yourself. The count will give you an even tempo.

STEP ONE: GENERAL HEAD MASSAGE

This not only promotes general relaxation and the harmonious flow of Qi and Xue, it is particularly good for those who are suffering from chronic sinusitis, respiratory allergies, TMJ, headaches, and anxiety or depression.

Massage the bridge of your nose on both sides with your middle fingers. Complete five circular rubbing motions moving from the top to the outside, down toward your nose, and then into the point above the inside corner of your eye.

Move your hands up from the bridge of your nose to the top center of your forehead.

Spread your hands apart with the fingers of your right hand moving down to the right temple and the fingers of your left hand moving down to the left temple. Massage the temple in a circular motion five times.

Move your hands up to top of head and bring them down to your neck. Rub the back of your neck up and down the tendons that extend on either side five times.

Move your hands to the outside of your neck until you can feel the lower point of your jaw joint. Rub that five times.

Now move your hands back to the bridge of your nose and in a smooth motion, trace the outline of your eyebrows to your temple and then move your hand down to the hollow of your cheek. Repeat this motion three times.

Slowly rotate your head, stretching your neck so your right ear is almost touching your right shoulder. Then slowly shift your head to the front so your chin is touching your chest. Then swing your head to the left so the left ear is almost touching the left shoulder. Now move it slowly toward the back. Look up at the ceiling. Repeat three times, then reverse direction and repeat again.

STEP TWO: EYE MASSAGE

In order to improve the circulation of Qi and Xue and improve visual clarity, you want to direct Qi to your eyes.

Place your index and middle fingers on the inside points of your eyebrows. Massage in a circular motion five times.

Move your fingers to the outer corner of your eyes and rub gently.

Move your fingers down from the corners of your eyes to the top of your jawbone. Then move the fingers slowly down the length of your lower jaw until they almost meet at your chin.

Place your palms together and rub them back and forth across each other until they become quite warm. Cup your hands over your eyes to share your hand Qi with them. Do not touch your eyes.

STEP THREE: GENERAL EAR MASSAGE

Use of general ear massage tonifies the whole body—every organ system, the joints and all body parts—and keeps hearing healthy.

Take your two middle fingers and gently rub around the entire ear several times.

Place your thumb inside your ear and your fingers along the widest part of the ear flap. Pull gently outward so the thumb moves from the inside to the outer edge of the ear. Hold for a count of three. Repeat three times.

Take each earlobe between your thumb and forefinger and rub gently, pulling downward.

Place your palms over your ears and massage the entire ear. Repeat five times.

Press your palms against your ears and then quickly remove your hands.

Shake out your hands and fingers. Sit quietly for two minutes.

STEP FOUR: NECK MASSAGE

This moves Qi and Xue along the spine.

Sit with your back straight and your head tipped ever so slightly forward.

Place your hands together in a prayer position. Open your fingers and allow them to interweave. Spread the palms apart so your fingers are lying across the backs of your hands and both palms are parallel to the floor.

Place your hands like a cradle against the back of your skull. Your thumbs should be pointing straight down on either side of your neck.

Massage the tendons beneath your thumbs from top to bottom. Repeat five times.

Raise your thumbs slightly to catch the point at the base of your skull where the bone meets the neck. Rub back and forth along this ridge. Go very slowly, probing the area, feeling where you want to apply more or less pressure. When you find the spot that is particularly tender to the touch, hold your thumb there for a slow count of six. Exhale while holding the point. Repeat as many times as you like.

STEP FIVE: TORSO MASSAGE

This step and the next are important for anyone who wants to keep the Lung System clear and the Heart Xue flowing smoothly. The steps are particularly helpful for digestive problems, asthma symptoms and congestion.

Moving your hands from your neck to the front of your body, glide them over your chest with long, smooth strokes of your open palms. Repeat several times.

Cross your arms. Using your first and second fingers, massage a point about two inches above the center of each nipple. Circle your fingers on the right hand over your left nipple; your left hand over your right nipple. You may feel your lungs open up.

Placing your palms flat on each side of your torso (left hand on left side, right hand on right side), move the Qi (from the point above your nipple that you just massaged) to the side and bottom of your lungs. Massage in a smooth, flat motion to the side of your torso and then down to your diaphragm.

STEP SIX: QI UP, QI DOWN

Place the tips of your fingers of your right hand on the pectoral muscle by the crook of your left arm.

Move your fingers in a circular motion, tracing a three-inch circle from the top of your chest, moving inward, down, to the outside and back up to the top. Repeat this, creating a spiral shape vertically down a line through the nipple. As you go in this direction (only!) move your hand down the full length of your torso.

Repeat the massage using the tips of your left-hand fingers on the right side of the torso. Make sure that you move your fingers from the top of your torso, toward your breast bone, then to your toes and finally toward your arm.

STEP SEVEN: ABDOMINAL MASSAGE

This technique is helpful for anyone with digestive problems, PMS, or cramps and helps harmonize the Large and Small Intestine, Liver, Spleen, Stomach and Gall-bladder. You way want to use oil infused with cinnamon to warm your belly if it is generally cold during your period or if you have loose stools and abdominal cramps due to cold.

Lie on a flat, firm surface. If needed, place a small pillow under your knees to take strain off your lower back.

Close your eyes halfway so there is less distraction. Inhale slowly and deeply.

Place your right palm on your stomach, above your navel, thumb lying against the skin pointing toward your chin. Place your left hand so it is on top of the right. Breathe in and out slowly, feeling the warmth under your hands. (If you are left-handed, place your left hand on your stomach first.)

Rub your stomach gently in a clockwise motion. Repeat twenty to forty times.

Raise your hands to the lower edge of your rib cage on either side of your torso. Smoothly massage down the length of your lower torso into the pelvic area and the groin. Repeat five times.

Now move your hand to the center of your abdomen, below your navel. Repeat motion as above.

Sit facing forward; inhale. Turn your head and neck but not your torso, and look over your left shoulder. Exhale. Now inhale as you turn your head and neck and look over your right shoulder. Exhale.

Take your right hand and place it along your waist on the left side of your body. Inhale. As you exhale slowly, move your palm forward along your waistline toward your navel. Reverse.

Now rub the front of your lower torso over your hip bones and down onto the tops of your thighs. Use one long, slow motion, with your palm open and flat.

Return to the first position, with your right hand over your stomach and your left hand on top of the right. Slowly, gently, rub in a clockwise motion for the count of six. Breathe in on the count of three and out on the count of six. Keep your eyelids at half-mast.

STEP EIGHT: CIRCULATING THE LOWER QI AND XUE

To promote harmonious flow of Qi and Xue, a complete massage keeps the motion going from your head through your feet in a complete cycle. (If you aren't going to give yourself a complete massage but are stopping after the abdomen, take time to do a couple of leg swings and stretches given in the Qi Gong exercise chapter on pages 153–166. If you are going to complete the massage cycle, remain seated with feet on the floor about eight inches apart.)

Sit on a firm, unupholstered, but comfortable chair without arms. Sit with good posture, but not stiffly. Rub the inner thighs with the same circular motion that you applied to the torso, always moving in a circle that goes from the top of the thigh (twelve o'clock), down the outside toward nine o'clock and up through six and three o'clock. Spiral down the thigh to the knee. Repeat three times.

Using your thumbs, press gently but firmly on the top center of the thigh and draw the thumb down to the knee. If you feel any tender spots, stop at that point and gently vibrate your thumb back and forth. Repeat three times.

When you come down to the top of your knee for the last time, hold your thumb in place and put your fingers across the center of the kneecap. Rub gently. Then rub your hands down the outside of your calf, from top to bottom (but not back up), five times.

Cross one leg over the other so your calf is in easy reach and lying parallel to the floor.

Place your fingers in the ridge that is formed between the near side of your shin bone and the calf muscle Slowly move them down from knee to ankle. Press with a firm, steady motion. If any point is tender, move your fingers in a circular motion on the point. Go from the top to the bottom. Repeat as desired.

STEP NINE: GENERAL FOOT MASSAGE

In Chinese medicine, the feet play a crucial role in the functioning of the channels. They are also associated with the harmonious balance of the Organ Systems and Essential Substances.

To help promote smooth flow of Qi and Xue and keep the channels working smoothly, you can give yourself a general foot massage, rubbing each part of the foot, starting with the ankle and ending with the toes. Devote extra effort to rubbing the toes and pay attention to the areas between the toes and between the long, thin bones that run along the top of the foot. Foot massage oil can provide an extra soothing touch: use peppermint-infused oil if you are hot and cinnamon-infused oil if you are cold.

As you rub your feet, you may want to target several acupuncture points for acupressure. Particularly important points to rub include Kidney 1, Spleen 4, Liver 3, and Gallbladder 41.

Kidney 1, directly in the center of each foot, right below the ball, is important to help keep the Kidney System working harmoniously, which impacts the functioning of all the other Organ Systems. Spleen 4, Liver 3, and Gallbladder 41 are also important foot points to help harmonize Qi and the Organ Systems.

STEP TEN: ARM AND HAND MASSAGE

After your arms and hands have worked hard massaging the rest of your body, it's their turn to be pampered.

An arm massage should be done from the shoulder to the tips of the fingers in long, slow strokes along the inside and the outside of the biceps and the forearm. Rub between or along bones, not on top of them.

After you extend the Qi through the arm, return to the acu-point, Large Intestine 14, at outside of the bicep below the armpit, the crook of the elbow, and the back of the wrist. On these points, press slowly and evenly. Breathe deeply.

A general hand massage can be done with the thumb moving in a gentle clockwise motion from the wrist to the fingertips, concentrating on the tissue between the bones and the areas around the knuckles and fingertips.

Once you've covered the entire surface of the hand, pull each finger out gently and rub the last section of your finger at the tip. Shake out the hands.

ACUPRESSURE MASSAGE

Acupressure massage uses the thumb and hands to stimulate the acupuncture points along the channels. In order to gain maximum effect without hurting yourself or straining your hand if you are massaging someone else, use the following guidelines.

Work the points with the soft, padded part of your thumb (where the thumbprint is).

Press down firmly and smoothly. Don't jab or stab at a point.

Always brace your thumb with the rest of your hand and fingers. For example, if you are massaging a point on your thigh, place your hand flat along the skin. Move your thumb into position, leaving the rest of your hand in contact with your leg. Press with your thumb. For more pressure or better leverage, don't pick up your hand. If you are massaging someone else, raise yourself up over them and press downward. If you are massaging yourself, lean into the pressure.

FOR ALERTNESS

Stomach 36 is located four finger widths from the hollow made when the knee is bent (below the kneecap) on the outside of the leg and one finger's width over from the crest of the shin bone. This point also is good for digestive problems, boosts energy, and helps strengthen the immune system. Stomach 36 was known in the old days as *three miles,* because when people hiked to the point of exhaustion, if they stopped and rubbed that point, they were able to go three more miles.

Large Intestine 4 is located in the webbing between the thumb and index finger. Press into the hollow against the bone from the index finger that extends down the length of the back of the hand. This is also good for any problems above the neck, such as sinus problems and headaches, and it is also beneficial for general inflammation, constipation, and diarrhea.

WARNING

Do not use Large Intestine 4 when pregnant.

FOR GENERAL HEALTH AND IMMUNE SYSTEM ENHANCEMENT

Stomach 36 is located four finger widths from the hollow made when the knee is bent (below the kneecap) on the outside of the leg and one finger's width over from the crest of the shin bone.

Large Intestine 4 is located between the thumb and forefinger in the middle of the forefinger bone that goes from the knuckle to the wrist.

Liver 3 is located at the point where the bones of the big toe and the second toe meet and form a V. The point is slightly in front of their junction.

Lung 7 is located one and a half inches above the transverse wrist crease on the back of the hand. It is above the large bump on the outside of the wrist bone.

Kidney 3 is located on the inside of the leg in the depression between the tip of the ankle bone and the Achilles tendon.

WARNING

During pregnancy, acupuncture should be received only from a practitioner skilled in management of pregnancy.

FOR LOW BACK PAIN

Kidney 3 is located on the inside of the leg in the depression between the tip of the ankle bone and the Achilles tendon. It is also good for immune enhancement.

Urinary Bladder 60 is midway between the ankle bone on the outside of the leg and the Achilles tendon, opposite Kidney 3.

Urinary Bladder 40 can be found in the center of the back of the knee. Points across the back of the knee correspond to the lumbar (lower back) vertebrae, so massage the entire crease. It is also good to massage down from UB 40 to UB 60.

Du 26 is located one-third of the distance below the nose, between the nose and the center of the top lip, in the slight indention. This is known as the emergency point and is used if someone loses consciousness. For acute back pain, stand up and hold on to the back of a chair with one hand. With the other, press relatively hard on the point with your fingernail while you move the back gently in and out of the area of pain by swaying your hips and torso.

Pericardium 7 is in the middle of the wrist crease on the inside of the arm. This point is also good for irregular heartbeat and tachycardia.

FOR GENERAL PAIN

Pericardium 6 is located on the inside of the wrist, three finger widths above the wrist crease, between the two bones. It is also good for anxiety, nausea, and morning sickness.

Pericardium 6 with Triple Burner 5 are known as regulating points and enhance overall calmness. Triple Burner 5 is located three fingers above the wrist crease on the top of the arm between the two long arm bones. Press TB 5 and P 6 at the same time for extra relief. This is good for carpal tunnel problems.

Ren 17 is located between the nipples at the center of the chest. It is used to release grief and improve breath by regulating Zong Qi. This endorphin point is the main point used to treat addiction.

Yintang is located between the eyebrows in the center of the bridge of the nose. It is used to ease pain and release tension, and is good for headaches and overall relaxation.

FOR SHOULDER

Triple Burner 4 can be found on the top side of the wrist at the midpoint of the wrist crease, between the two arm bones.

Triple Burner 5 is three finger widths above the wrist crease on the top of the arm between the two arm bones.

Small Intestine 3 is located in the indentation below the little finger knuckle on the outside of the hand. It is good for neck and shoulders. If you have a stiff neck, rotate your neck in and out of the area of stiffness while pressing the point. It is also good for clearing the brain.

FOR THE MID-BACK

Liver 3 is located at the point where the bones of the big toe and the second toe meet and form a V. The point is slightly in front of their junction.

Gallbladder 40 is in the hollow indentation just to the front of the outside ankle bone.

FOR GYNECOLOGICAL PROBLEMS

Spleen 6 is located four finger widths above the tip of the inside ankle bone, behind the shin bone.

Ren 4 and 6: divide the line that runs from the navel to the pubic bone into five equal sections. Ren 4 is three sections below the navel; Ren 6 is one and a half sections below the navel.

DEEP TOUCH HEAD MASSAGE

To ease tension, calm the Shen and stimulate the harmonious flow of Xue, you may want to focus on a head massage. Use your two middle fingers. Always move your hands upward and to the outside, down to the low point and then upward along the inside. This massage is also effective for smoothing out wrinkles produced by tension.

Wash the face with mild cleansing solution and, if you like, apply a gentle cream or oil that will not irritate the eyes.

Begin on the eyebrows (point 1) and run your thumbs slowly and evenly the length of the brow from the inside to the outside.

Move to the lower orbit and rub around each eye, along the bone, moving from the outside, underneath, to the inside, and then the top of each eye.

On the cheek, target the four points on the diagram above and gently move your fingers out from those points to the edge of your ears. Repeat five times.

On your jaw in front of your ear at Stomach 7, rub downward to Stomach 6 and then along the jawline to your chin. Repeat three times.

Massage each ear by starting at the lobe and working your way around the rim, moving into the center, and then back out to the rim.

Move your two middle fingers to the center of your forehead at the hairline. Rub your right hand clockwise and your left hand counterclockwise.

Move to the neck at GB 20 and UB 10 (see diagram for locations). Press gently and firmly on those points for the count of five. Release. Rub with your fingers flat, moving your hands in a circular motion.

Moving your hands around to the top of your shoulder blade (GB 21 and TB 15), rub smoothly and deeply.

Lie back with eyes closed and keep your breathing slow, steady, and deep.

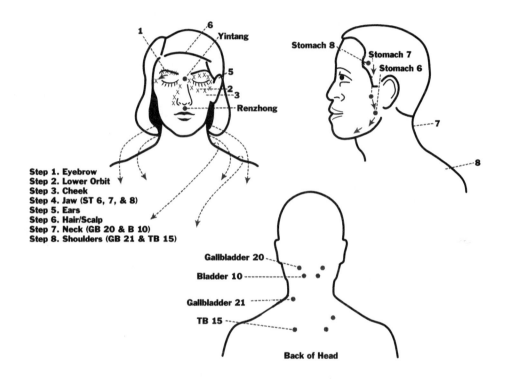

1
6 Yintang
5
2
3
Renzhong

Step 1. Eyebrow
Step 2. Lower Orbit
Step 3. Cheek
Step 4. Jaw (ST 6, 7, & 8)
Step 5. Ears
Step 6. Hair/Scalp
Step 7. Neck (GB 20 & B 10)
Step 8. Shoulders (GB 21 & TB 15)

Stomach 8
Stomach 7
Stomach 6
7
8

Gallbladder 20
Bladder 10
Gallbladder 21
TB 15

Back of Head

LOWER BACK SELF-MASSAGE

Much low back pain comes from Qi Stagnation and constricted muscles and tendons. This massage allows you to gently stretch them out and ease discomfort.

Sit on a chair with your feet flat on the floor about six inches apart.

Inhale. Roll your chin down to your chest as you exhale. Bend your back and drop your shoulders forward as you inhale. Continue downward until your chest is resting on your thighs as you exhale.

Make two fists. Bring your hands up behind your back.

Make circles with your hands all over your lower back.

Press deeply along your spine as far up as you can reach.

Pound lightly with fists along your lower back, hips, and on either side of your spine. To increase the benefits, use the pounding motion to massage Large Intestine 4, an acu-point that is located in the webbing between the thumb and the index finger. Stimulating this point helps invite the low back pain to move downward from the back and to disperse.

Let your arms and hands dangle at your sides.

Slowly roll back up, using your arms to help by walking them up your legs. Keep your chin tucked in and your upper back rounded until you are sitting upright. Then let your spine straighten from the bottom up.

AMAZING EAR MASSAGE

If the eyes are the windows to the soul, then the ears are the road maps. Located in the external part of those two little organs are acu-points that provide a direct route to all the important functions of the mind/body/spirit.

Many of the acu-points are more potent than points located on the channels; for example, the three no-smoking points, known as the Shenmen, the Sympathetic, and the Lung, are much more effective in promoting nicotine detoxification than any other acu-points on the body.

To rub ear points, you may use your finger, a cotton swab, or you can purchase an ear massage probe at a natural health store. Don't worry about touching other points. You'll be able to tell when you're in the right position: ear points become very sensitive and tender when there is a disharmony in the corresponding part of the body.

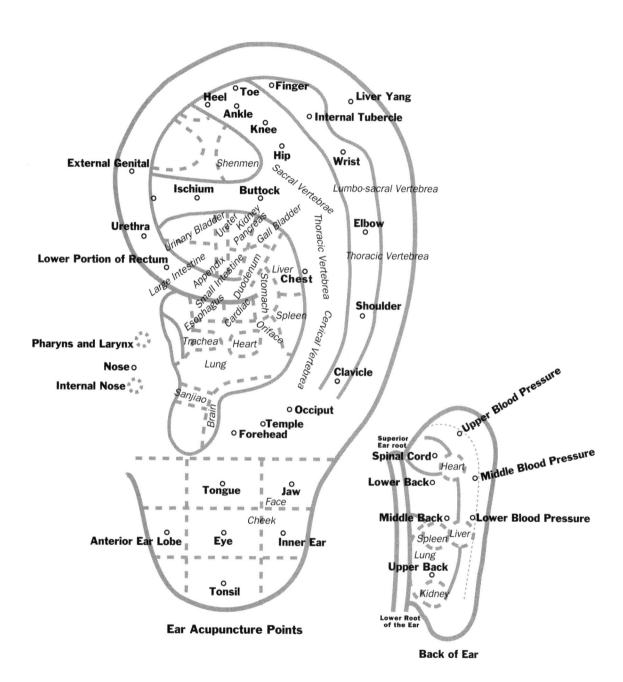

Ear Acupuncture Points

Back of Ear

Anatomical Portion of the Ear	Name of Point	Action/Indication
	Middle ear	Hiccups, jaundice, symptoms of digestive system, and skin
	Lower portion of the rectum	Constipation, anus prolapse, external and internal hemorrhoids
	Urethra	Frequent urination, retention of urine, painful urination
Helix crus and helix	External genitalia	Inflammation of external genital organs, eczema of the perineum, impotence
	Anterior ear apex	External and internal hemorrhoids
	Ear apex	Fever, hypertension, inflammation of the eyes, painful diseases
	Liver Yang	Liver Qi stagnation, liver Yang preponderance
	Helix 1–6	Fever, tonsillitis, hypertension

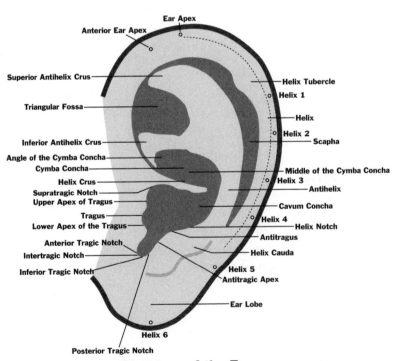

Structure of the Ear

Anatomical Portion of the Ear	Name of Point	Action/Indication
	Finger	Pain and dysfunction in finger(s)
	Interior tubercle	Expelling wind and stopping itching
	Wrist	Pain and dysfunction at wrist
Scapha	Elbow	Pain and dysfunction of elbow
	Shoulder	Pain in the shoulder
	Clavicle	Pain in the clavicle and peripheral arthritis of the shoulder
	Toe	Pain in the toe(s)
Superior antihelix crus	Heel	Heel pain
	Ankle	Ankle sprain, pain and dysfunction in corresponding body part
	Knee	Pain and dysfunction of the knee, such as a sprain, and arthritis of the knee joint
	Hip	Pain in hip
Inferior antihelix crus	Buttocks	Pain in buttocks
	Ischium	Sciatica
	End of the inferior antihelix crus	Antispasmodic and analgesic, nourishing the Yin and Yang; indications: pain of internal organs, palpitations, spontaneous sweating, night sweats, functional disorders of the autonomic nervous system
Antihelix	Cervical, thoracic, and sacral vertebrae	Pain at the corresponding part of the spine
	Neck	Strained neck, pain or dysfunction of the neck
	Chest	Pain or stuffiness of the chest or pain in the chest area
	Abdomen	Abdominal or gynecological diseases, lumbago

Anatomical Portion of the Ear	Name of Point	Action/Indication
	Shenmen	Sedation, easing addiction withdrawal symptoms, restoring peace of mind, relieving pain, clearing heat
Triangular fossa	Triangular depression	Gynecological diseases, impotence, prostatis
	Superior triangle	Hypertension
	Superior tragus	Ear disease, dizziness, and vertigo
	Nose	Nasal obstructions and other nose problems
Tragus	Supratragic apex	Reducing heat and relieving pain
	Infratragic apex	Reducing heat and relieving pain, antispasmodic
	Pharynx-larynx	Acute and chronic laryngitis and tonsillitis
	Internal nose	Allergic rhinitis and other nose diseases
	Antitragic apex	Asthma, bronchitis, parotitis, itching skin
	Middle border	Incomplete mental development, enuresis
	Occiput	Sedation and pain relief, headaches, insomnia, dizziness
Antitragus	Temple	Sedation and pain relief
	Forehead	Sedation and pain relief
	Brain	Mental deficiency, insomnia, dream-disturbed sleep due to Kidney deficiency
	Mouth	Facial paralysis, inflammation of the mucous membranes of the mouth
	Esophagus	Difficult swallowing, dysfunction of the esophagus
	Cardiac orifice	Indications, gastritis, gastroduodenal ulcer, and other diseases and symptoms of the gastric region

Anatomical Portion of the Ear	Name of Point	Action/Indication
	Duodenum	Duodenal ulcer, pylorospasm
	Small Intestine	Indigestion, palpitations
	Appendix	Appendicitis, diarrhea
	Large Intestine	Diarrhea, constipation
	Liver	Liver Qi stagnation, eye disease, and disorders on the sides of the lower abdomen
Cymba conchae	Pancreas	Migraine, diseases and symptoms of the bile duct, pancreatitis
	Kidney	Nephritis, lumbago, tinnitus, impotence
	Bladder	Lower back pain, sciatica, cystitis, enuresis, retention of urine
	Angle of cymba conchae	Prostatitis
	Middle cymba conchae	Low fever, abdominal distention, impaired hearing, parotitis, mumps
Cavum conchae	Heart	Insomnia, palpitations, hysteria, night sweats, angina
	Lung	Cough and asthma, skin diseases, hoarse voice, all addiction withdrawals, anesthesia point
	Trachea	Cough and asthma
	Spleen	Diarrhea, chronic indigestion, abdominal distention, functional uterus bleeding
	Triple burner	Removing obstruction from water passages, clearing up heat, and stopping itching
	Intertragus	Skin diseases, impotence, irregular periods, dysfunction of endocrine system, menopausal symptoms
	Frontal tragic notch	Glaucoma, pseudomyopia, and other eye diseases
	Lower tragic notch	Hypotension

Anatomical Portion of the Ear	Name of Point	Action/Indication
Ear lobule	Back tragic notch	External eye inflammations
	Cheek	Facial paralysis and other facial problems
	Tongue	Glossitis
	Jaw	Toothache, submandibular arthritis
	Section 4 of earlobe	Toothache and lethargy due to emotional responses
	Eye	Acute conjunctivitis, myopia, other eye diseases
	Internal ear	Tinnitus, auditory vertigo, impaired hearing
	Tonsils	Acute tonsillitis
	Upper root of auricle	Headache, abdominal pain, asthma
	Lower root of auricle	Headache, abdominal pain, asthma
Back auricle	Groove of inferior helix crus	Hypertension, skin diseases
	Heart	Insomnia, dream-disturbed sleep, hypertension, headache
	Spleen	Abdominal distention, diarrhea, indigestion
	Liver	Distention and fullness of the chest area, soreness and aching of lower back
	Lung	Asthma, digestive disorders and diseases, fever
	Kidney	Headache, dizziness, vertigo, irregular periods

Adapted from *Chinese Acupuncture and Moxibustion,* Foreign Language Press, Beijing,1987

SHIATSU PARTNERED MASSAGE

Japanese Shiatsu works by exerting deep pressure on the acupuncture points of the body and can be used to harmonize the Essential Substances and the Organ Systems as well as to relieve muscle pain and tension. The Shiatsu touch is explained on page 173.

The following massage cycle provides a complete stimulation of all the channels.

You may extract sections from it to address specific body parts or enjoy the whole. A complete massage should take about fifty minutes. When you're through, you'll discover that it is as beneficial for the person doing the massage as the person receiving it.

Proper breathing is important for both the person giving and receiving the massage. Long, slow breaths with even slower exhalations help tranquilize the mind/body/spirit and assist in the smooth flow of Qi.

Have the person receiving the massage lie on his or her stomach on a comfortable but firm surface such as an exercise mat or plush carpet. Do not do this massage on a bed or standard massage table.

BEGIN MASSAGE

The one who's giving the massage kneels at the person's left side, waist high.

SPINAL STRETCH

Place your right hand on the lower back of the person with your fingers pointing toward the toes. Place your left hand on the upper part of the back, with the heel of your hand just below the vertebra that protrudes below the bottom of the neck at the top of the spine.

Gently rock the body from side to side. Then, holding your right hand in place, stretch the spine upward by softly applying an upward pressure to the heel of your left hand. Continue gently rocking the body as you stretch the spine.

Now move your hands so that your right hand is on the person's right hip and your left hand on the left shoulder blade. Stretch and rock. Then reverse sides and repeat.

Move the left hand, palm down, to the area between the shoulder blades and place your extended right hand, palm down, on top of the left.

Raise up slightly on your knees for more leverage and begin pushing around— but not directly on—the spine as you move your hands down toward the lower back. Work down to the tailbone and back up.

Leave your left hand between the shoulder blades and place your right hand on the tailbone and do another spinal stretch while gently rocking the body.

LEG STRETCH

Have the person adjust his or her legs so the toes are pointing slightly inward. Place your left hand on the back of the right leg along the crease between the thigh and the buttock. Cup your right hand over the right heel. Stretch the leg and rock it gently. Repeat on the left leg. Again, raise up on your knees if you need more leverage or to apply more pressure.

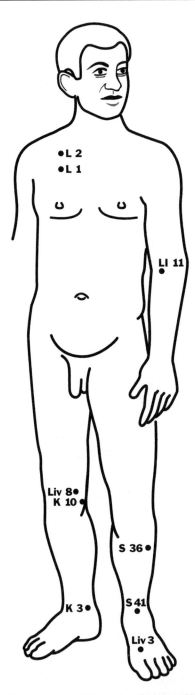

Acupressure Points for Shiatsu Massage

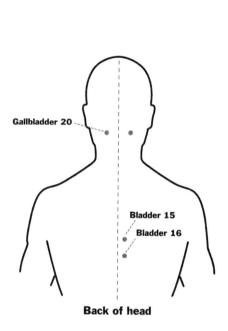

Gallbladder 20

Bladder 15

Bladder 16

Back of head

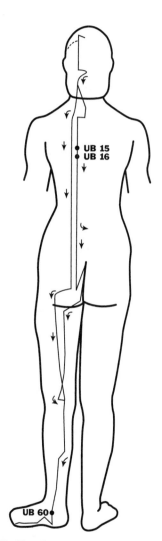

UB 15
UB 16

UB 60

The Bladder Channel of Foot-Taiyang

BACK TO THE BACK

Now the one giving the massage should stand up and straddle the person, placing the feet alongside the person's hips and facing forward. Never sit on the person; it constricts blood flow and tightens muscles. Bending over the person, use both hands to press down on the area just to the right and the left of the spine. Don't press directly on the spine. Work the inner and outer Urinary Bladder channel (see page 187).

Now slip hands under the person at the hip bones and gently raise him or her up a little bit off the floor. Release, and then press down gently on the sides of the back up from the hip bone.

Use your thumbs, supported by your fingers, to press and release as you massage out from the spine over the back above the hip bone.

Move your thumbs to press along the length of the tailbone. Then go to the buttocks and smoothly press along the outside, the middle, and the inner section of each cheek from the lower back to the top of the thigh.

Take a break, shake your hands, and do several shoulder shrugs.

ARM MASSAGE

Move the person's left hand up behind him or her so the back of the hand is resting against the lower back.

Take your thumbs and, beginning with the lower back, press them into the area between the spine and the ribs. Move up toward the left wing bone. Press with your thumb or thumbs in the area below and under the wing bone. Slip the edge of your hand under the bone and pull the wing bone up and out.

Find the point in the middle of the wing bone where there is a slight indentation. Press firmly but gently on that spot.

Move the person's left arm so it is horizontal to the body and holding the wrist in both hands, gently pull the arm out from the shoulder, shaking it slightly. Let the arm lie flat, extending in a comfortable position out from the body.

Massage the upper left arm, using both your hands. Then hold the left wrist in your left hand and use your right thumb to massage down the Triple Burner channel (see page 27). Then use your thumbs to work on the Large Intestine channel (see page 23).

Bend the arm and locate Large Intestine 11 at the spot on the outside of the arm where the crease from bending the elbow ends (see page 140). Massage. Then work down the forearm with both your hands.

Flex and extend the wrist. Work Large Intestine 4, the fourth point up from the tip of the index finger (see page 140).

Turn the person's hand over, and using both your thumbs, rub the palm of the hand from below the fingers to the wrist.

Pull and slightly twist the fingers.

Shake out the wrist and arm.

Move to the right side of the person and repeat on the other arm.

LEGS AND FEET

Kneel at the person's left side. Make sure his or her toes are pointed slightly inward.

Put your left hand under the person's right knee and lift it up slightly.

Place your right hand flat on the back of the knee and press gently, massaging the crease at the back of the knee.

Work the right calf with both hands, combining your thumbs and the flat of your hand.

Concentrate on Kidney 3, Urinary Bladder 60 (see pages 186 and 187).

Lift the leg and support the knee while turning the foot out. Place your right hand on the person's ankle. Use the left hand to rub the length of the Gallbladder channel between muscle and bone along the outside of the leg.

Then stretch the calf with one hand on the back of the knee, the other on the heel.

Switch to the other leg.

Sit cross-legged at the person's feet and place the feet in your lap.

On the right foot, press on Kidney 3 and UB 60 (see pages 186 and 187). Then work the heel with both your thumbs and move down the center of the foot, through the arch. Stop at the big toe and massage the area and Stomach 41 (see page 186). Move to the top of the foot and work the spaces between the bones and tendons, Liver 3. Massage the toes and pull them out gently from the foot.

Rotate the foot to stimulate the ankle. Then slap the bottom of the foot and stretch the foot one more time. Let the foot rest gently on the mat.

Do the other foot.

SHOULDER AND NECK LIFT

Have the person flip over on to his or her back. Place a small pillow under the person's knees to ease the tension on the small of the back, if necessary. Kneel or sit cross-legged at the person's head.

Place your hands under the person's shoulders along the shoulder blades.

Draw the fingers of your left hand up along the person's spine to the head. Hold the head with your fingers resting on the bony ridge at the top of the neck and the base of the skull.

Use your right hand to massage the neck.

Rub UB 15, UB 16, and GB 20 with the left hand and thumb at the base of the skull (see page 187).

Cradle the person's head in both your hands and turn it slowly from side to side and back and forth. Ask the person to inhale deeply. Then, as he or she exhales, take the head and neck and ever so gently move it up and forward, stretching the back of the neck and moving the chin onto the chest. Release down slowly and carefully. Repeat.

HEAD, EARS AND FACE

With the head resting on the mat, move your hands to the ears and begin scratching lightly all around and behind. Then use your thumb and index finger to work the ear from the outer rim into the well. For more extensive ear massage information, see pages 178–184.

Move to the scalp, rubbing vigorously. When you are finished, pull the hair gently.

Place one hand under the head, holding the lower part of the skull. Place the other so it is grabbing the chin. Gently pull the head out from the neck. Hold for a few seconds. Release gently.

For detailed face massage, see pages 168, 169 and 170.

ABDOMEN

Rub the Ren channel (also called the conception vessel) starting at Ren 17 on the breastbone between the nipples (see page 31). Move to the ribs above the breastbone, using your thumbs to move from the center outward on both sides of the chest. Work Lung 1 and Lung 2 (see page 186).

Rub the stomach above the navel with both hands going clockwise. Use a rocking motion, alternating between the fingers and the heel of your hand.

Move your hands down to the area below the navel. Focus on Ren 4 and Ren 6 (see page 31).

Hold your hands about one to two inches above the hara (or dan-tien) area. Feel the flow of energy.

LEGS

Sit along the left side of the person. Starting at the top of thigh, take the left leg in both your hands and work your thumbs down the leg toward Stomach 36 (see page 186).

Bend the person's left leg and draw his or her knee over toward your lap. Do not force it.

Use both hands and thumbs to work the Liver channel that runs along the inside of the leg. Work Liver 8 and Kidney 10 along the calf.

Straighten the leg out and squeeze along the top of the thigh to the knee.

Massage the kneecap.

Move both your hands alongside the shin bone, working the points on either side of it from the knee to the ankle.

Repeat on other leg.

FINISH

Help the person sit up. Stand behind him or her so your knees support the back.

Lean over and work your thumbs into the tops of the shoulders. Remember to brace your thumbs with your hands; don't jab. Then squeeze along the shoulders, working from either side of the neck out to the shoulders and down the arms, squeezing all the time.

Pound the back and shoulders with your fist or open hand.

Breathe deeply, shake out your hands. Say thank you to the person.

WESTERN MASSAGE TECHNIQUES

SELF AND PARTNERED HAND MASSAGE

Hand reflexology is a Western form of hand massage that correlates specific parts of the hand to internal organs and body parts as they are described in Western medicine. All hand massage can be done to yourself or by a partner.

To massage your hand using reflexology points, identify the location of your disharmony or disease in terms of Western anatomy and find the corresponding

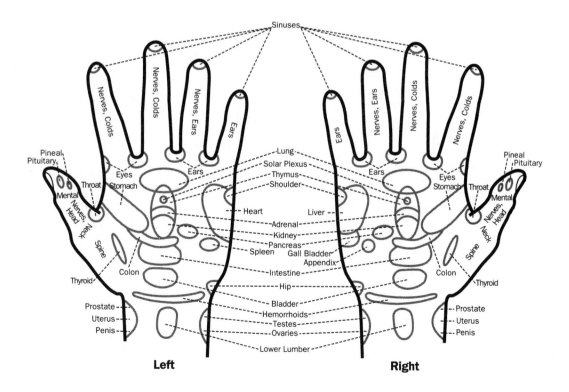

area for that body part on the chart. If you hurt your knee jogging, use the hip and knee area on the chart; if you have irritable bowel syndrome, use all the colon areas; if you have headaches, use the head area on the chart; if you have uterine cramps, use the womb area on the chart.

Use your thumb to rub the appropriate spot and your fingers to hold the hand firmly but gently. Press with your thumb(s) gently until you feel a sensitivity, pain, or tenderness. Using the flat part of your thumb, draw it across the spot, rotating it gently in a clockwise motion. To use two thumbs, place them side by side on the appropriate area of the hand and draw them out and down in opposite directions, rubbing one in a clockwise and one in a counterclockwise motion.

SELF AND PARTNERED FOOT MASSAGE

Reflexology also has a system of foot massage that has identified specific points on the foot correlating to specific internal organs and parts of the anatomy.

To massage your foot using reflexology points, use the same technique as described above for hand reflexology.

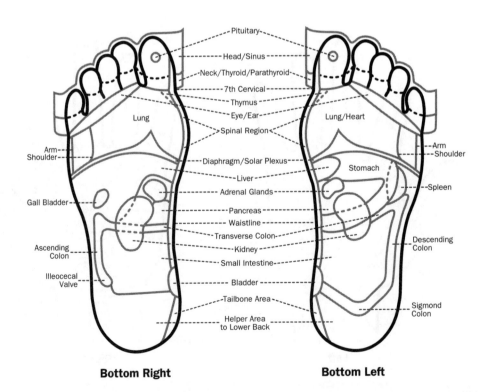

Bottom Right   **Bottom Left**

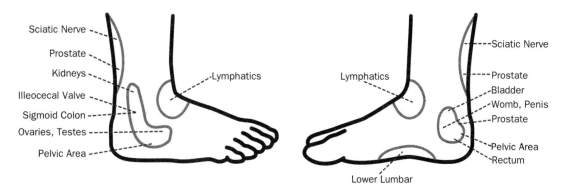

COOL SAUNAS AND HOT SOAKS AND COMPRESSES

Cool saunas and hot soaks and compresses can stimulate the flow of Qi and Xue and can dispel Cold and Dampness. These immersion therapies should not be assaults on your body, making you turn beet red, sweat profusely, or become overheated. Instead, they should be gentle persuaders that soothe the Shen and calm the mind. They are often used to increase the effectiveness of acupuncture, massage, and herbal therapy.

Soaks

You may soak your whole body by slipping into a deep tub of water or just dip your hands or feet into a basin. In general, you should soak for no more than thirty minutes to avoid dehydration. Always drink lukewarm herb tea or room-temperature water while soaking. When you get out of a soak, it is important to use a plant-based cream, oil, or moisturizer to seal the skin and prevent dehydration and flakiness. Avoid mineral oils and those that are full of dyes, preservatives, and artificial colors and aromas.

General Calming Soaks   These soaks are designed to calm the Shen and pacify the Heart.

LATTE DELUXE
1 tubful of hot water
2 cups to 1 quart of whole milk (organic, if possible)
4 cinnamon sticks

Fill the basin or tub to the top with water from 100–110°F, depending on your comfort level. You will have to decide what feels good to you.

Stir in 2 cups to 1 quart whole milk (chemical free).

Drop in a bag made of unbleached cheesecloth filled with broken cinnamon sticks. Eliminate the cinnamon if you have heat-related problems or very sensitive skin.

Soak for 20–30 minutes.

SLEEP-EASE

1 tubful of warm to hot water
1 cup loose chamomile or ½ cup chamomile and ½ cup valerian
1 large square unbleached cheesecloth
1 piece of natural twine

Place 1 cup of loose chamomile tea or ½ cup chamomile and ½ cup valerian
    on a square of unbleached cheesecloth and tie it into a ball, securing it with
    a piece of natural twine.
Fill a basin or tub with water. Select a temperature that feels relaxing to you.
Place the cheesecloth bag in the tub of water and steep for ten minutes.
Soak yourself for 20–30 minutes.

To Stimulate Qi and Dispel Cold

GINGERBATH

1 tubful of warm to hot water
1 cup grated or sliced fresh ginger
1 large square of unbleached cheesecloth
1 piece of natural twine

Grate 1 cup of fresh ginger onto a square of cheesecloth and tie it into a ball,
    securing it with a piece of twine.
Fill your basin or bath with medium hot water.
Place the cheesecloth bag in the tub of water and steep it for 10 minutes.
Soak yourself for 20–30 minutes.

ROSEMARY RUSH

1 tubful of warm to hot water
½ cup fresh rosemary
1 large square of unbleached cheesecloth
1 piece of natural twine

Place ½ cup fresh rosemary in a natural cheesecloth bag.
Steep the bag in a basin or tub of hot water for 10 minutes.
Soak yourself for 15–30 minutes.

LEMONADE

1 tubful of warm or cool water
Four lemons

Fill the basin or tub with either warm water (100°F) or cool water (90°F).

Squeeze the juice of four fresh lemons into the water. Now slice the lemons
into thin rounds and drop them into the tub.
Soak yourself for 20–30 minutes. Rinse your skin in warm water.

THYME AND AGAIN
1 tubful warm to hot water
2–5 drops thyme oil

Place a few drops of thyme oil in a hot bath. (Follow instructions on bottle;
intensity of oil varies.)
Soak yourself for 20 minutes.
Rinse your skin in cool water.

To Dispel Heat

PEPPERMINT COOLER
½ gallon of peppermint tea made with ½ cup fresh peppermint (or other edible
fresh mint)
1 tubful of cool water

If you can buy or grow fresh peppermint, that is the best. Boil ½ cup in a gallon
of water for 10 minutes.
Draw a cool bath and add the boiled peppermint tea, strained, to the tub.
Slip in and soak yourself until you begin to feel cool. Don't wait until you are
cold.
If peppermint is not available, use spearmint instead.

To Fight Pernicious Influences The following soak may trigger detoxification
reactions, such as achy sensations and irritability. These are natural reactions and
are nothing to worry about.

BLEACH BATH
½ to 1 cup Clorox liquid bleach
1 tubful of hot water

Only Clorox brand bleach is recommended. If you are doing the cleansing diet
you may want to do these two together.
Add Clorox to a hot bath (as hot as you can stand without feeling faint) and
soak yourself for twenty to thirty minutes.
Shower after bathing to make sure you don't leave a trail of bleach on your
carpet or have bleach residue on your skin.
Only do one soak a week.

SUPER HOT TUB
1–5 pounds of Epsom salts
1 tubful hot water

This is a strong cleansing bath.
Fill tub with water as hot as you can stand.
Add Epsom salts.
Soak for 10–15 minutes. If you get dizzy at any point, get out of the tub.
Two baths a week are effective for muscle relaxation and detoxification.

SALTY DOG
1 pound sea salt
1 pound baking soda
1 tubful hot water

Add sea salt and baking soda to hot bathwater.
Soak for 10–15 minutes.
Two baths a week are effective for muscle relaxation and detoxification.

HERBAL FOOT REST
½ cup yarrow root
1 basin boiled water

Steep yarrow in boiled water.
After 5–10 minutes, it should be cool enough to slip your feet into the water.
Soak feet for 20 minutes.

To Ease Dryness   Prepared herbal oils are available that can soothe or stimulate and keep your skin supple and smooth. They are a bonus for the senses when added to your soak. Choose those that appeal to your senses.

Cool Saunas

Saunas can hit a devastating 108° to 112°. In Chinese medicine, these temperatures are understood to create disharmony and cause Qi Deficiency. In Western terms, they are hard on the heart and skin and the immune system. Cool saunas, on the other hand, offer many benefits. They cleanse the skin (the largest organ in the body in Western terms), ease nasal congestion, and help the body to detoxify through the skin.

Set the sauna temperature for 102°F. When your skin becomes moist and you feel warmed throughout, gently scrub the skin with a loofa or a soft bristle brush. This gets rid of dead skin and excreted toxins.

Compresses

Warming compresses have the advantage of being able to deliver concentrated heat or cool and herbal infusions directly onto the spot that needs the attention. They are recommended for chronic and acute stomach problems, gynecologic discomfort, headaches, strains, and sprains. These are the ones we suggest you can do at home. There are others that your practitioner may prescribe, depending on your constitution and the presence of any disharmonies.

Hot Spots   These compresses are to dispel Stagnant Qi, Cold and Dampness.

GINGERLY
⅓ large gingerroot, grated or finely chopped
1 square unbleached cheesecloth
2 quarts boiled water

Place grated ginger in a square of cheesecloth and tie it securely.
Place cheesecloth bag in pan with 2 quarts water. Boil for 10 minutes.
Remove cheesecloth bag from water and set aside.
Soak a washcloth in the ginger brew and apply over the troubled area.
Repeat until you feel warm and more comfortable.

QUIET COUGH
Make a compress as above, substituting peppermint leaves for ginger.
Apply compress to upper chest.
Breathe in the peppermint aroma.

To Cool a Fever   Place 4 drops of eucalyptus oil on a washcloth saturated with cool water. Place on chest. Breathe deeply. Repeat until body temperature feels lower.

In addition to these homemade compresses, your practitioner may prescribe special herb compresses for problems such as eczema, psoriasis, acne, bruises, pain, and swelling. There are also ready-made compresses, such as Hydrocollator packs, that you heat in a pot of boiling water, microwaveable packs that mold to your neck or shoulders, and herbal packs that become moist when warmed.

PART THREE

Where the Paths Meet: Comprehensive Healing Programs to Maintain and Restore Wholeness

CHAPTER TWELVE

Introduction to New Medicine's Comprehensive Programs of Healing

The following comprehensive programs are designed to be used as a guide for your own self-directed healing. They bring together basic Chinese medicine therapies with other healing arts so you can maintain harmony and treat disharmony in your mind/body/spirit. They are offered to you as plans that you can follow or adopt to suit your personal needs.

Maria is a client who aggressively followed her own comprehensive plan and created an enormous difference in her life. When she came to the clinic in June 1994, she was complaining of chest pain, incredible fatigue, and low-level depression. She was so incapacitated that she had to take a leave of absence from her job as a registered nurse.

After examining her, I suspected she might have hepatitis and suggested she go immediately for a blood chemistry test that would reveal her liver functions. I needed to know liver enzyme levels and to have them retested throughout treatment so I could follow the reduction in liver inflammation and shape acupuncture therapy to address the changing symptoms of the disease. This is another example of how important it is for Chinese and Western medicine to work together. Each therapy helps the client forge the most effective treatment possible.

The results of Maria's blood work showed she had elevated liver enzymes and hepatitis C.

Immediately she began searching the medical literature to find out about the disease and treatment options. She said to me, "I'm in charge here. What I want are your suggestions."

I recommended she see a liver specialist for a consultation. Again, it's important that the client receive information about options from Western and Eastern practitioners. The doctor said he could offer her only one possible remedy, interferon, which she knew had only a 10 to 20 percent success rate and even then was only effective for a couple of years. It didn't seem worth the possible side effects. She refused. Her liver doctor agreed to monitor her while she pursued other therapies.

She started with a regular regime of herbs, four times a day. She also had others for use when certain symptoms would flare up. She received acupuncture twice a week and followed a strict self-care program of dietary therapy and moxibustion. In addition, she found she was beginning to examine her life from a spiritual side, seeking to eliminate high stress. She began practicing Qi Gong and meditating. "I'll follow the whole regime for the rest of my life," she says. "It's improved my liver function and my spirit and mind. I'm clearer and more centered."

When she had her blood work in June of 1994, two liver enzymes—SGOT and SGPT—were high. After four months of herbal treatments, she was retested. "Those enzymes dropped forty-seven and fifty-nine points," she recalls. "The doctor was very impressed. In fact, he tested me three times to make sure of the results. I did stop drinking during that time, and that might account for a ten-point drop, but not fifty-nine points. And it's only gotten better. The last time I had liver pain was March of '95.

"If I met someone who was sick, and couldn't find a solution, I'd tell that person to try Chinese medicine and other forms of alternative healing. It doesn't hurt, it's not real expensive, and it's working."

If you're ready to follow Maria's lead and try a comprehensive program, you may select the general program for basic good health and a strong immune system; the stress and depression management program; the women's gynecologic health program that includes special sections on PMS and menopausal symptoms; the digestive disorders management program; or the addiction detoxification program.

Each one contains a section on self-care therapies including Chinese dietary therapy; Qi Gong exercise and meditation; acupressure, massage, and reflexology; and soaks and compresses. There's also a section on assembling a healing team of health care providers, including Chinese medicine practitioners, standard Western doctors, and a variety of Eastern and Western healers.

CHAPTER THIRTEEN

Strengthening Organ Qi and Protective Qi

A Comprehensive Program for Basic Good Health and a Strong Immune System

The New Medicine offers each of us the opportunity to resist disease by strengthening the basic energy of the body.

Combining Chinese medicine's ability to reinforce our Organ Qi and Protective Qi so
the immune system can resist assaults by bacteria and viruses;
+
Western medicine's diagnostic technology and helpful medications;
+
Alternative therapies, such as Yoga, Shiatsu, homeopathy, Ayurvedic medicine,
chiropractic, Western herbs and aromatherapy,
=
New Medicine's program for becoming noticeably healthier and stronger.

PART ONE: SELF-CARE: A SEVEN-STEP PLAN FOR STAYING HEALTHY

STEP ONE: DAILY LOG

The core of every comprehensive plan is the daily log. It allows you to keep track of your physical and emotional actions and reactions for one to two weeks.

As a result, you will become conscious of the relationship between your daily habits and the way you feel in mind/body/spirit. That may indicate areas of your lifestyle that you want to change in order to strengthen your Organ and Protective Qi and your immune system.

These changes should be gradual. It's not necessary—in fact it's not good for you—to make swift and extreme shifts in the way you live, your diet, or your activities. You want to allow your body and your consciousness to grow so that you are comfortable with the changes you make.

Keeping the Log

To keep a log, buy a small notebook that you carry around with you, in your pocket or tote. You can then give a copy of this self-contained record to your practitioner and Western doctor and keep one for yourself.

1. Make note of everything you eat and when you eat it. Don't leave out that afternoon glass of juice or a late-night snack.
2. Write down how much physical activity you get, both formal exercise and in doing your daily chores or job.
3. Keep track of your sleep patterns: when you go to sleep, if you awake during the night, and how long you sleep. Include information on snoring, night sweats, tingly limbs, nightmares, and dreams.
4. List how much you drink, including sodas, coffee, tea, alcohol, and sugared drinks.
5. Note the time of day you experience any changes in your blood sugar level, such as a sinking feeling, overwhelming fatigue without other causes, headache, a funny taste in your mouth, inability to concentrate, or a craving for sweets.
6. Keep a record of your digestion, elimination, and urination. Note times you feel hungry, bloated, gassy, constipated, have loose stools, acid indigestion, etc. Also note how often you urinate and what color it is.
7. Record any prescription, over-the-counter, or recreational drugs that you take. Make note of the quantity and your reaction both during and after the initial sensation. If possible, note why you took that particular drug.
8. Write down your emotions throughout a day including grogginess or grumpiness in the morning (before you have coffee), highs and lows, feelings of depression, happiness, calmness, anger, frustration, etc. Try to pinpoint the times they occur and the triggers, if you know.
9. Make note of your mental acuity—when you feel clear or unclear.

STEP TWO: IMPLEMENTING A DIET PROGRAM

Using Information from Your Daily Log

Reviewing your log, look for recurring symptoms of disharmony associated with your diet.

• Do you become bloated, gassy, tired or grumpy after eating a particular food?
• Notice foods that you eat frequently, foods that you crave and those that you avoid. Can you associate those with physical symptoms of disharmony or mood changes?
• Do your symptoms of disharmony change depending on your meal schedule?
• Do your food-related symptoms change depending on what time of the month it is?

• Is there a correlation between your eating patterns, the amount of alcohol or caffeine you drink and any symptoms of disharmony?

Once you've examined your daily log for these and other associations between diet and well-being, you may target certain eating habits that you'd like to change—at least temporarily—to see if they eliminate troubling symptoms of disharmony in your mind/body/spirit.

A Cleansing Routine

Now that you've identified those elements of your diet that may be diminishing your ability to fight off disharmony and disease, you may want to give your body a little break. A cleansing diet removes irritants and toxins and soothes the system. The First-Step Diet Therapy program (chapter 7, page 95), can last from one day to one week. If you feel weak or unable to do a phase, you may skip it or shorten it.

Using the Power of Food

As you build a new approach to your diet, you want to harness the power of food. Chinese medicine considers diet to be the first line of defense against disease, and Western medicine is discovering new evidence almost daily of the relation between nutrition and disease prevention. This association between food and general health is the result of what the Chinese call *Energetics*—the power within food that **cools or warms** the metabolism and Organ Systems, **moisturizes or dries** the Organ Systems, and **increases or decreases** the flow of Qi, Jing and Xue. Keeping Energetics balanced is essential to maintain harmony in Organ Qi and Protective Qi.

In order to protect the Energetics in the food you consume, eat as much organic foods and hormone- and antibiotic-free meats as possible. Drink only filtered water or spring water to eliminate sources of bacteria, protozoa, and other organisms now commonly found in municipal water systems. It is important to use a water filter that eliminates all organisms. Reduce fat intake to between 20 and 30 percent of calories.

A Balanced Diet A balanced diet delivers the right mix of Energetics. It includes warm foods and doesn't contain too many raw foods. For most healthy people, a three-meal-a-day plan offers the best sustenance. Breakfast should provide a moderate amount of whole grains and protein. Cooked, warming foods stimulate the Qi. Lunch should be the largest meal of the day, with a wide variety of vegetables, fruit, grains, legumes, and a small amount of meat protein, if desired. For dinner, the smallest meal of the day, you want to avoid stimulating foods such as proteins and spicy food.

Your daily calorie intake should include 75 percent of calories from grains, vegetables, and legumes. Grains should account for two-thirds of this and vegetables and legumes for the other third. Fruits should constitute about 10 percent of your daily calories, and dairy and protein, including meats, should add up to about 10 percent.

Food Tonics

Therapeutic foods that combine Energetics with herbal action provide a tonic for the Qi and Xue. Once a week, eat a serving of San Qi Chicken, Dang Gui Chicken or a congee made with American ginseng, codonopsis, or red dates. (For recipes, see pages 97–102.)

For more information on how diet can increase your immune strength and maintain a well-balanced constitution, refer to chapters 6 and 7.

STEP THREE: IMPLEMENTING AN EXERCISE/MEDITATION PLAN

Exercise/meditation is as important to a preventive health program as sound nutrition. Not only does it keep all the Essential Substances in harmony and nourish the Organ Systems, it soothes the Shen and keeps the mind clear and alert. To help you figure out how you can use exercise/meditation in your preventive health care program, refer to your daily log.

First, make note of those days you do exercise: what form, for how long, and how you felt before and after. Were there some forms of exercise that made you feel better than others? Did you feel better exercising for a shorter or longer length of time?

Next, see if there is a correlation between anger, depression, or stress-related moods and maladies and your exercise schedule. Are you tenser when you don't exercise? Do you have more symptoms of disharmony after you don't exercise for a while? Does exercise exhaust you and make you feel blue?

Although each person should exercise to suit his or her Qi, so that neither Qi Stagnation nor depletion is encouraged, a generally well-balanced weekly routine

SUGGESTED WEEKLY EXERCISE/MEDITATION ROUTINE

Day 1	Day 2	Day 3	Day 4	Day 5	Day 6	Day 7
15 minutes Qi Gong warm-up (page 159) 30 minutes aerobics of choice 15 minutes cool-down and meditation	1 hour Qi Gong full routine (begins on page 159) or Yoga	30 minutes aerobics 30 minutes weight-bearing exercises	1 hour Qi Gong full routine (begins on page 159) or Yoga	30 minutes aerobics 30 minutes weight-bearing exercises	15 minutes Qi Gong warm-up (begins on page 159) 30 minutes aerobics of choice 15 minutes cool-down and meditation	Rest

may incorporate a minimum of twenty minutes of exercise/meditation a day. One hour of exercise and meditation, four to six days a week, is optimal. The exercise should be a blend of aerobic movement such as jogging, cycling, tennis, swimming and step classes, as well as Qi Gong, weight-bearing exercises, stretching exercises including Qi Gong and Yoga, and breathing and meditation exercises.

STEP FOUR: USING SOAKS, SAUNAS AND COMPRESSES

Saunas, soaks and compresses are all effective ways to calm the Shen and keep the Qi and Xue flowing harmoniously. See chapter 11 for details on how to use them for preserving your health.

Once a week take a twenty-minute sauna at 102° F and/or a soak to help ease stress and eliminate Dampness and Excess. Soaks to stimulate Qi are recommended if you've had a sedentary week.

STEP FIVE: USING MASSAGE AND MOXIBUSTION FOR SELF-HEALING

Moxa and many massage techniques can help maintain Organ System harmony and strengthen Protective Qi. Read through chapter 11. All the various massages will benefit your health and harmony. For attention to particular trouble spots, use your daily log as a guide to the type of massage that will benefit you the most. Notice if you have a recurring complaint about neck, shoulder or back pain try the routines on pages 170 and 174–177 or if you are bothered by pain with your monthly cycle try page 178. For a complete body massage and general Qi harmony, do the ten-step Qi Gong self-massage (page 168), and to ease discomfort, try the partnered Shiatsu massage on page 184.

Other generally tonifying massages include acupressure, moxibustion and ear massage.

Acupressure can calm or invigorate and ease tension. For a listing of acu-points you can self-massage and the symptoms they address, see page 173. Of particular benefit in a general program are Kidney 3, Ren 4 and Ren 6. Follow the acupressure techniques described for these points on pages 31 and 186. Repeat as often as desired. **Ren 6 should not be used during pregnancy.**

Moxibustion should be a regular part of your tonification routine. Use moxa on Stomach 36 one to seven times a week. Once a week, enjoy Spleen 6, Ren 6, and Ren 12. Ren 4 and Ren 6 are particularly beneficial for women who may have a tendency toward cold. Gallbladder 39 is especially good for anemia and is often used for people with chronic immune function. For details on how to use moxibustion, see page 148. And for location of the points see the illustrations on pages 31, 140–144 and 186–187. **Ren 6 and Spleen 6 should not be used during pregnancy.**

Ear massage can soothe the whole body. For general well-being, sit in a quiet room. Close your eyes and breathe evenly. To begin a general ear massage, using a gentle rubbing and pulling motion, start with the outer fold where it attaches on the top front of the ear and move slowly around the rim, into the inner cavities, and end with the earlobe. The process should take about two to three minutes. Repeat on the other ear. You may also target specific Organ Systems for reharmonizing. The ear massage chart and instructions are on pages 178–184. Massage points called Shenmen, Lung and Spleen are recommended for overall rebalancing.

STEP SIX: NUTRITIONAL SUPPLEMENTS

Follow the general supplement plan on page 111 that includes an all-purpose vitamin and mineral supplement. Additional vitamin E and beta-carotene are advised, as is a regular dose of *Lactobacillus acidophilus.* This maintains digestive flora that are destroyed by antibiotics, hormones, and a poor diet. Don't take large doses of any supplement without the advice of a practitioner, doctor, or nutritionist.

Sean came to the clinic because of his allergies after he had given up on standard Western treatments. That was four years ago. "Taking a chance on a new kind of medicine seemed risky then, but I felt like it was riskier not to take the chance. And it turned me around," he says.

Over time, Sean's exposure to another way of thinking about maintaining wholeness produced even greater changes. He began to meditate, improved his diet and continued regular acupuncture and herbs, when needed.

After some soul-searching, he gave up his high-stress job and developed his own business. He also does improvisational theater—a lifelong dream. Layers of stress and stress-related disharmonies fell away. Not only did he change how he thought about his health care, he changed how he thought about himself as a whole person.

"When everything they were doing for me made me feel so much better, I got some confidence in myself. I mean, I started thinking I could probably take pretty good care of myself . . . or find people who could help me do it."

Today, he is healthier in mind/body/spirit. "As it was happening, all the changes seemed the most natural thing in the world. But looking back, I see I've come a long way."

STEP SEVEN: THE WELL-STOCKED MEDICINE CABINET

In order to treat colds and flu, minor cuts and stomach upset, you want to stock the most effective Chinese and other natural remedies. In this medicine cabinet you will find, in addition to Chinese first aid, several homeopathic medicines for acute problems. For constitutional problems, I don't prescribe homeopathic medicine; I refer clients to a homeopathic practitioner. But for acute problems, I often suggest that clients purchase the products listed below.

All the suggested Chinese and Western remedies are generally safe, but they should not be used by children under twelve or the elderly without the advice of a practitioner.

THE MEDICINE CABINET

Indications	Formula	Ingredients	Suggested Use and Dose	Suppliers
Colds, flu	Isatis Gold™	Goldenseal Echinacea Isatis extract	Colds and inflammations with fever, including flu and bronchitis 3 tablets every 2–4 hours until symptoms are relieved (discontinue after 48 hours if no results)	Health Concerns
	Loquat Cough Syrup (chuan bei pi pa gao)	Pi Pa Ye (eriobotryae) Bei Mu (fritillaria) Sha Shen (glehnia) Wu Wei Zi (schizandra) Chen Pi (citrus peel) Jie Geng (platycodon) Ban Xia (pinellia) Bo He (herba menthae) Kuan Dong Hua (tussilago) Xing Ren (semen armenica) Feng Mi (honey)	Expectorant for dry cough 10 cc 2–3 times per day	Chinese herb store
	San She Dan (Chuan Bei Lu) cough syrup	Snake biles Fritillaria Semen armenica Asarum etc.	Cough with phlegm One small vial 2–3 times per day	Chinese herb store
Digestive distress **Stomach flu** **Food poisoning**	Curing/Konning Pills (pill curing)	Tian Ma (gastrodia) Bai Zhi (rx. angelica) Ju Hua (chrysanthemum) Bo He (herba menthae) Ge Gen (pueraria) Tian Hua Fen (trichosanthes) Cang Zhu (atractylodes) Yi Mi (semen coix) Mu Xiang (saussurea)	For nausea and diarrhea associated with stomach flu or food poisoning 1/2 to 1 small vial 2–3 times a day or as needed for 3–5 days	Chinese herb store

Indications	Formula	Ingredients	Suggested Use and Dose	Suppliers
		Hou Po (cortex magnolia) Ju Hong (pericarpium citrus) Huo Xiang (agastaches)		
	Quiet Digestion™	Fu Ling (poria) Yi Yi Ren (coix) Shen Qu (shen chu) Hou Po (magnolia) Bai Zhi (angelica) Cang Zhu (red atractylodes) Mu Xiang (saussurea) Huo Xiang (pogostemon) Gu Ya (oryza) Tian Hua Fen (trichosanthes) Ju Hua (chrysanthemum) Chi Shi Zhi (halloysite) Ju Hong (citrus) Bo He (mentha) Mai Ya (malt)	For gastric distress, including abdominal pain, sudden and violent cramping, abdominal distention, nausea, vomiting; also treats gastro-enteritis, motion sickness, hangover, and jet lag **Do not use if appendicitis is suspected** 1–3 pills 2–3 times a day or as needed for 3–5 days, after or between meals	Health Concerns
Sinus congestion	Pe Min Kan Wan	Cang Er Zi (xanthium) Huo Xiang (pogostemon) Ye Ju Hua (wild chrysanthemum) Bai Zhi (rx. angelica) Xin Yi Hua (magnolia flower)	For runny or stuffy nose, rhinitis, sinusitis, sneezing 3–4 pills as needed Use no more than 1–3 days without consulting practitioner Do not use if pregnant without consulting practitioner Contains animal products	Chinese herb store

Indications	Formula	Ingredients	Suggested Use and Dose	Suppliers
	Bi Yan Pian	Cang Er Zi (xanthium) Xin Yi Hua (magnolia flower) Gan cao (licorice) Jie Geng (platycodon) Wu Wei Zi (schizandra) Lian Qiao (forsythia) Bai Zhi (rx. angelica) Zhi Mu (anemarrhena) Ye Ju Hua (wild chrysanthemum) Fang Feng (siler) Jing Jie (schizonepeta)	Acute and chronic rhinitis, thick mucus with headaches 3–4 pills as needed	Chinese herb store
	White Flower Oil (for external use only)	Menthol Wintergreen oil Camphor (Some brands also include eucalyptus oil)	Stuffy sinuses due to allergy, colds, or chronic sinusitis Use one drop in steaming water for sinus steaming (turn off water from a boil **before** steaming) Be careful not to burn eyes—oil is very strong	Chinese herb store
Trauma, acute injury, bruising	Yun Nan Pai Yao	San Qi (radix pseudo-ginseng)—main ingredient	Acute injury, bruising, bleeding 1/8 of a bottle of the powder with warm water or wine every two hours after an acute trauma **The red pill is for emergency use only** 1–2 pills from the blister pack every 2 hours	Chinese herb store

Indications	Formula	Ingredients	Suggested Use and Dose	Suppliers
			If internal bleeding is a possibility or bleeding does not stop, call a doctor immediately	
	San Qi 17™	San Qi Myrrh Frankincense Calamus Curcuma Persica Dang Gui Red peony Sappan wood Cinnamon twig Kadsura Acronychia Eupolyphaga Carthamus Rhubarb Tsou-Ma-Tai Licorice	For traumatic injuries, bruising, pain 2–3 pills three times a day If internal bleeding is a possibility or bleeding does not stop, call a doctor immediately	Seven Forests
	Dr. Shir's Liniment™ (external use only)	Alcohol Rhubarb Safflower Myrrh Arisaema Persica Mastic Dang Gui Bone Powder Turmeric Camphor	Pain and swelling of acute or chronic soft tissue injuries Lightly rub liniment on affected area as needed Do not use on open wounds **For external use only**	Spring Wind
	Zheng Gu Shui (external use only)	San Qi (radix pseudoginseng) Bai Zhi (rx. angelica) Ji Gu Xiang (cinnamomum camphora) Bo He Nao (menthol extract)	Pain due to fractures, ligament tears, muscle sprains, and bruising Lightly rub liniment on affected area as needed	Chinese herb store

Indications	Formula	Ingredients	Suggested Use and Dose	Suppliers
		Zhang Nao (camphora crystals) Wu Ma Xun Cheng (croton tiglium) Qian Jin Ba (moghania) Da Li Wang (inula cappa)	Do not use on open wounds **For external use only**	
Pain	Yunnanpaiyao	San Qi (radix pseudoginseng) main ingredient	Pain due to acute injury, bruising, bleeding 1/8 of a bottle of the powder with warm water or wine 2–3 times a day Use for 2–3 days **The red pill is for emergency use only**	Chinese herb store
	Channel Flow™	Corydalis extract Angelica Peony Cinnamon twig Dang Gui Salvia Myrrh Frankincense	Abdominal pain, especially menstrual pain, or fibromyalgia 2–4 pills three times a day for	Health Concerns
For massage	Po Sum On	Peppermint oil Dragon blood Cinnamon oil Scutellaria Tea oil Licorice	This oil tends to be cooling—used generally for people with hot conditions Apply a few drops of oil and massage skin; or apply to a towel with warm water and lay on neck and shoulders; also used for steaming	Chinese herb store

Indications	Formula	Ingredients	Suggested Use and Dose	Suppliers
	Warming Oil	Cinnamon-infused oil	This oil is warming; use to increase circulation or to warm an area Use for full body massage or for area massage such as for feet or abdomen	KW Botanicals
	White Flower Oil	Menthol Wintergreen oil Camphor Some brands also include eucalyptus oil	This oil is cooling and is best to use for very small areas—good for sinus massage and on bruises Apply a drop or two to the affected area and lightly rub	Chinese herb store
	Moxa Stick	Chinese mugwort Sometimes other herbs are added	Can light the stick and burn over an area that has been injured, including bruises, sprains, strains Not for use over areas that have open sores, cuts, or are bleeding Use for 5–10 minutes until the area is warm and pink Take care not to burn yourself (See p. 148 for instructions on use of moxibustion)	Chinese herb store

NON-CHINESE MEDICINES

Indications	Formula Name	Ingredients	Suggested Use and Dose	Suppliers
Stress, traumatic incident	Rescue Remedy (Bach flowers)	Star of Bethlehem Rock rose Impatiens Cherry plum Clematis	A few drops under the tongue after a traumatic event	Health food store
Trauma, acute injury	Arnica Salve (homeopathic)	Homeopathic arnica in an oil base	Rub onto area of sprain or soreness during the first 24–48 hours	Health food store Pharmacy
	Arnica Pills 6x or 30x (homeopathic)	Homeopathic arnica	Take a few tablets under the tongue every 1–3 hours depending on severity of injury	Health food store Pharmacy
Digestive distress, nausea, morning sickness	Ginger Tea (home brewed)	Fresh gingerroot (also is a Chinese herb)	Use for nausea without burning sensation 2–3 slices fresh ginger boiled for ten minutes in 1 cup water Every 2–3 hours or after meals	Grocery store
Colds, influenza	Oscillococcinum (homeopathic)	Anas barbariae Hepatis et cordis extractum HPUS 200CK Sucrose Lactose	Several tablets under tongue every 1–3 hours depending upon severity of symptoms	Health food store Pharmacy
	Echinacea tablets or tincture	Echinacea purpura	For beginning stages of colds and flu See instructions on particular brand	Health food store Pharmacy
Skin inflammation	Calendula Salve (homeopathic)	Homeopathic calendula	Use for minor skin irritation **Do not use if there is a break in the skin**	Health food store

---

THE HEALTHY TRAVELER

Traveling can cause all kinds of disharmonies, but you can protect yourself with a few easy-to-follow routines.

For Jet Lag

Before you go

Begin overcoming jet lag with the diet outlined in Dr. Charles Ehret's book, *Overcoming Jet Lag*, three days before you depart. I've found it works to eliminate jet lag even after long flights.

Melatonin, the natural hormone that controls the body's clock, is available over the counter. Taken at night for two days before you leave and for two days upon arrival, it helps adjust your sleep cycle.

On the plane

Drink a glass of water every hour you're in the air to avoid dehydration and constipation.

Avoid alcohol or caffeine, which make dehydration worse.

Eat small, light meals when flying, or follow Dr. Ehret's jet-lag diet.

Exercise on the plane by getting out of your seat and walking around at least once an hour.

Qi Gong exercise is also possible, particularly the exercises where you visualize your muscles tensing and relaxing (see page 159). Some airlines offer in-the-seat aerobics on long flights.

On arrival

Take Curing Pills (see the Medicine Cabinet) once a day for three days.

Take melatonin for two days after arrival. Do not use for more than a total of four days, since the long-term side effects are unknown.

Acupuncture treatments soon after arrival can reharmonize your system quickly.

For Digestive Problems

Changes in water, stress, time changes, and bacterial infections can all contribute to digestive problems when you travel. Take *Lactobacillus acidophilus* before leaving home and continue during your travels. At the first sign of cramping or diarrhea take Curing/Konning Pills. (See the Medicine Cabinet.)

PART TWO: ASSEMBLING YOUR HEALING TEAM

When you're putting together a healing team for a preventive health care program, you want to blend the contributions of Eastern and Western practitioners. Although I practice Traditional Chinese Medicine, I occasionally employ homeopathic remedies for acute conditions such as sprained ankles, bruises and the flu, and I prescribe Bach flowers for stress-related disorders. I often refer clients to other practitioners, such as Western doctors, chiropractors, and massage therapists, for treatment. For more detailed information on these other healing arts, see the resource section in the back of the book or your local library or bookstore.

Your Chinese practitioner can provide regular checkups, offer advice on management of common colds and flu, administer preventive acupuncture and herbal therapy, help you develop a dietary and exercise/meditation routine that is tailored to your individual needs, and help you maintain harmony of Shen and work to rebalance your Essential Substances and Organ Systems before they develop full-blown disharmonies. The practitioner should become familiar with your constitution and medical history so diagnosis is as accurate as possible.

Your Western practitioner may provide yearly diagnostic testing and a baseline evaluation. The yearly exam may include a Pap smear for all women over sixteen, mammograms for women over forty, screening for sexually transmitted diseases, exams for intestinal and prostate cancers at appropriate ages, skin cancer checkups, and cholesterol and cardiovascular monitoring.

Alternative practitioners who specialize in homeopathy, chiropractic, Ayurvedic medicine, Shiatsu, or other healing modalities are an important part of a preventive program. The key is to tell each member of your healing team about the various treatments you are receiving.

INTEGRATING VARIOUS THERAPIES

There are a few guidelines that you may want to follow so that your eclectic approach doesn't create disharmonies either in your mind/body/spirit or among your various practitioners.

Don't put off seeking a standard Western medicine baseline examination. Western medicine provides many important healing tools, from surgical procedures to life-saving antibiotics and diagnostic procedures. Using these modalities within the context of Chinese medicine is the best way to reap Western medicine's benefits and minimize its risks. For example, if you have a systemic infection from a wound, refusing antibiotics could lead to death. However, antibiotics also cause all kinds of systemic problems and overdependence has led to bacterial mutations that antibiotics cannot kill. Chinese medicine, if used along with antibiotic therapy, can remove the negative systemic side effects such as yeast overgrowth and bowel disturbances and can decrease the long-range need for antibiotics.

In short, Western medicine understands how to treat specific, narrowly defined health problems. Chinese medicine offers the opportunity to improve the strength and health of the whole body so that specific problems can be resolved. That's why New Medicine places such an emphasis on using all other modalities in the context of Chinese medicine.

Always inform all practitioners of the various healing arts that you are using. Share the results of your Western examinations (and evaluations from other health care providers) with your Chinese medicine practitioner. The tests may help guide treatment, and in the case of serious illness, may allow the Chinese medicine practitioner, Western doctor, and other caregivers to work together to provide the best care possible.

Don't use yourself as a guinea pig. Seek the guidance of a trained practitioner if you have any questions, and don't hesitate to get a second opinion on any health-related matter. Remember, you're the captain of your health care team.

Don't mix drugs and/or herbal medications without the advice of a trained practitioner. When seeking advice on herbal medications, ask a Chinese herbal practitioner, not someone who has no training in the contraindications or possible side effects.

BEGINNING THE COMPREHENSIVE PROGRAM

Step One: Obtaining a Western Baseline

It's important to rule out cancer and other life-threatening problems and to identify an illness that can be treated quickly and effectively by Western medicine. Western doctors recommend the following baseline and diagnostic tests.

Tests	Ages 19–39	Ages 40–64	Ages 65+
Health checkups	Annually	Annually	Annually
Blood pressure	Every 2 yrs.	Every 2 yrs.	Every 2 yrs.
Breast self-exam	Monthly	Monthly	Monthly
Breast exam by doctor	Every 1–3 yrs.	Annually	Annually
Cholesterol screening	Every 1–5 yrs.	Every 1–5 yrs.	Every 1–5 yrs.
Mammography		Every 1–2 yrs. to age 50, then annually	Annually
Pap smear	Every year	Every year	Every year
Stool test for occult blood		Annually after age 50	Annually
Sigmoidoscopy		Every 3–5 yrs. after age 50	Every 3–5 yrs.
Tetanus-diphtheria booster	Every 10 yrs.	Every 10 yrs.	Every 10 yrs.
Flu shots			Annually

Step Two: Obtaining Chinese Medicine Diagnosis and Treatment

When you go to a Chinese practitioner, it's important to establish communication between the Chinese and the Western doctor. Both practitioners should be aware of what you are doing as director of your own healing process.

At the Chinese practitioner, you can expect to be treated with acupuncture, moxibustion, and herbs.

Acupuncture and Moxibustion For maintenance when you are experiencing no troublesome disharmonies, you should receive an acupuncture treatment with the change of each season. The fluctuations in humidity, temperature, diet, amount of sunlight, and physical activity that happen from season to season make it helpful to get your Qi rebalanced quarterly. The points that would provide strengthening include Large Intestine 4, Lung 7, Stomach 36, Kidney 3, Liver 3, and Spleen 6.

For most people, however, more frequent and more specific treatments may be recommended. Very few of us are so perfectly balanced that we don't have some complaint or could not improve upon our ability to fight off disease. The best acupuncture schedule can only be determined through individual diagnosis by your practitioner.

Herbs The basic preventive health care routine is a blend of herb soups and congees and, if your practitioner suggests, a low dose of the immune-strengthening formula Enhance™ (see page 220) if you are susceptible to colds and other viruses. When you feel as if you are getting a cold or flu, you may use Cold Free™ and Isatis Gold™ (see Medicine Cabinet, page 208) to relieve the onset of symptoms. However, the practitioner will evaluate you according to traditional diagnosis and most likely provide a formula for whatever specific pattern and symptom-sign complex you may have.

Step Three: Bringing in Other Modalities

Most people will benefit from a monthly Shiatsu massage, visits to the chiropractor when muscle tension or soreness causes alignment problems, nutritional counseling from a Western, macrobiotic, or Ayurvedic nutritionist, and exposure to any other Eastern healing traditions including Tibetan medicine or Yoga.

WHEN THE IMMUNE SYSTEM IS WEAKENED

A comprehensive program of preventive health care is effective for those whose mind/body/spirit is in fairly good harmony. Unfortunately, people may be hit with unexpected assaults on their harmony, such as a car accident or serious illness, or they undermine their naturally strong constitution by living with chronic stress or emotional upheaval, using drugs or alcohol and engaging in excessive or unsafe sex. They become easy targets for viruses, bacteria and other organisms.

However it happens, when the body is attacked and the immune system weakened, people need extra strong therapy to maximize their strength.

If you have an immune-related disease such as herpes, chronic fatigue, chronic hepatitis, or are HIV positive, a combination of aggressive Chinese and Western therapy can provide far-reaching benefits. I have developed a therapeutic approach to managing such immune-related syndromes that relies on newly created herb formulas, traditional Chinese acupuncture and moxibustion treatments, and West-

Formula	Herbs in Formula	Chinese Function	Western Diagnosis
Enhance™*	Ganoderma (Ling Zhi) Isatis Extract (Ban Lang Gen/Da Qing Ye) Millettia extract (Ji Xue Teng)	Tonifies: Qi, Xue, Yin, Yang, Jing	Decreased cellular immunity or humoral immunity
	Astragalus (Huang Qi) Tremella (Bai Mu Er) Andrographis (Chuan Xin Luan) American Ginseng (Xi Yang Shen) Hu Chang (Hu Chang) Schizandra (Wu Wei Zi) Ligustrum (Nu Zhen Zi) White atractylodes (Bai Zhu) Cooked rehmannia (Shu Di Huang) Lonicera (Jin Yin Hua) Salvia (Dan Shen) Aquilaria (Chen Xiang) Curcuma (Yu Jin) Epimedium (Yin Yang Huo) Viola (Zi Hua Di Ding) Oldenlandia (Bai Hua She She Cao) Citrus (Chen Pi) Cistanche Rou Cong Rong White peony (Bai Shao) Lycium fruit (Gou Qi Zi) Ho Shou Wu (He Shou Wu) Laminaria (Kun Bu) Eucommia (Du Zhong) Tang-Kuei (Dang Gui) Cardamom (Sha Ren) Licorice (Gan Cao)	Clear Heat/Clean Toxin Clears Phlegm Strengthens: Wei Qi, Spleen System, Stomach System, Kidney System	Frequent colds and flu HIV/AIDS Chronic fatigue immune dysfunction syndrome (CFIDS) Chronic viral illnesses associated with immune dysfunction

*Developed by Misha Cohen

ern therapy. The detailed scope of these programs will be discussed in an upcoming book. For those who are interested in finding out about the research that's been done on using Chinese therapy in conjunction with Western treatments for immune-related disease and the names of Chinese herbal formulas used specifically for immune enhancement, see the reference section.

COMPREHENSIVE PROGRAM FOR BASIC GOOD HEALTH AND A STRONG IMMUNE SYSTEM

Seven-Step Self-Care Plan	
Self-monitoring	**Keeping the Log** The daily log should make note of your diet, physical activity, and body rhythms, including sleep, elimination, emotional changes, and mental acuity.
Implementing a dietary program	**Step 1. Using information from your daily log.** Reviewing your log, look for recurring symptoms of disharmony associated with your diet. **Step 2. A cleansing routine.** The first-step diet removes irritants and toxins and soothes the system. **Step 3. Using the power of food.** As you build a new approach to your diet, you want to harness the Energetics of food. **Step 4. Establish a balanced diet.** Your daily calorie intake should include 75 percent of calories from grains, vegetables and legumes (grains should account for $2/3$ of this and vegetables and legumes for the other $1/3$). Fruits should be about 10 percent and dairy and protein—including meats—should add up to about 10 percent. **Step 5. Food tonics.** Use therapeutic foods that combine Energetics with herbal action to provide a tonic for the Qi and Xue.
Implementing an exercise/ meditation plan	Use your daily log to help you structure a plan that suits your constitution. The exercise should be a blend of aerobic movement such as jogging, cycling, tennis, swimming, step classes, and Qi Gong; weight-bearing exercises; stretching exercises including Qi Gong and Yoga; and breathing and meditation exercises.
Using massage and moxibustion for self-healing	Moxa and many massage techniques can help maintain Organ System harmony and strengthen Protective Qi.
Using soaks, saunas and compresses	Saunas, soaks and compresses are all effective ways to calm the Shen and keep the Qi and Xue flowing harmoniously.
Nutritional supplements	Follow the general nutritional supplement plan. Additional vitamin E and beta-carotene are advised, as is a regular dose of *Lactobacillus acidophilus*.

Assembling the Healing Team	
Obtaining a Western baseline	It's important to rule out cancer and other life-threatening problems and to identify an illness that can be treated quickly and effectively by Western medicine. Regular diagnostic and screening tests are recommended. This information and information about any ongoing Western treatment should be presented to your Chinese medicine practitioner.

Obtaining Chinese medicine diagnosis and treatment	When you go to a Chinese practitioner, it's important to establish communication between the Chinese and the Western doctor. Preventive routine: Acupuncture, Moxibustion, and Herbs
Bringing in other modalities	Most people will benefit from a monthly Shiatsu massage, occasional visits to the chiropractor, nutritional counseling from a Western, macrobiotic, or Ayurvedic nutritionist, and exposure to any other Eastern healing traditions including Tibetan medicine and Yoga.

CHAPTER FOURTEEN

Calming the Shen

A Comprehensive Program for Easing Stress, Anxiety and Depression

In Chinese medicine, the mind/body/spirit is understood to be one entity. A peaceful mind and spirit are inseparable from the health of the body. A healthy body is part and parcel of a balanced mind and spirit. Depression, anxiety and stress-related disorders are not singled out as symbols of an embarrassing failure of character, as they so often are in Western cultures. Instead, they are seen as a manifestation of a network of responses that are physical, spiritual and psychological.

This expansive view of the origins of what the West calls mental illness is just beginning to be accepted by Western doctors and scientists. Now, for example, depression is no longer seen as a linear result of bad thoughts or weakness. In a feedback loop reminiscent of Chinese medicine's concept of the role of Yin/Yang, depression is seen as a manifestation of outside stimuli, emotional reactions to that stimuli, brain chemistry, and genetic predisposition all working together to produce the disharmony that is identified as depression.

Blending the newest Western insights and the traditional Chinese therapies, the New Medicine offers a four-pronged approach to managing depression, anxiety disorders and stress.

STEP ONE: SELF-CARE TO CALM AND STRENGTHEN THE MIND/BODY/SPIRIT

Shen imbalances are usually caused by internal emotional disharmonies (traumas such as abuse and neglect) and by suppression of emotions (caused by denial and inability to contend with or express feelings). They are often associated with Qi Stagnation and disharmony in the Heart and Liver Systems.

There are two types of Shen imbalances: *Disturbed Shen* and *Lack of Shen*. Disturbed Shen causes forgetfulness, disorientation, memory lapses, insomnia and lackluster eyes. Extreme disharmony is associated with madness. Lack of Shen is associated with a flat affect and inability to communicate. Lack of Shen makes a person seem as though, "The lights are on, but no one's home."

Alcoholism, depression, chronic headaches, digestive disturbances, panic attacks, anxiety, schizophrenia and psychosis are all the manifestations of various degrees of Shen imbalance.

Any program to ease Shen imbalances focuses on restoring harmonious flow of Qi and Xue and balancing the Heart and Liver Systems.

Dietary Guidelines

In addition to following the basic guidelines for sound nutrition set out in chapter 6, those suffering from Shen imbalances should eat certain foods to regain harmony.

Eat foods that regulate or move Stagnant Qi and motivate stuck energy: basil, bay leaves, beets, black pepper, cabbage, chicken livers, coconut milk, garlic, ginger, kelp, leek, nori, peaches, scallions, and rosemary. Avoid alcohol, fatty foods, food additives, unnecessary medicines, and overindulgence in sweets.

Eat foods that sedate excess Liver conditions: beef, chicken livers, celery, kelp, mussels, nori, and plums. Avoid coffee, fried foods, excessively spicy foods, heavy red meat, sugar, and sweets.

Eat foods that help ease Xue Deficiency: oysters, sweet rice, liver, chicken soup, Dang Gui Chicken (see recipe on page 99.) Avoid raw fruit and vegetables, cold liquids or ice.

Exercise/Meditation Guidelines

Qi Gong exercise and meditation is tremendously effective in soothing the Shen and balancing the flow of Qi and Xue. A daily routine that includes at least twenty minutes of Qi Gong exercises and twenty minutes of meditation can help ease anxiety, stress, and depression almost immediately. See page 159 for the basic Qi Gong routine.

In addition, studies have repeatedly shown that aerobic exercise has a positive effect on people suffering from chronic depression. Although initial motivation may be difficult because of Qi Stagnation, the effort is vastly rewarding. Any aerobic activity, from walking to swimming or cycling is suitable, depending on your level of fitness. One half hour every morning, in addition to the Qi Gong, is recommended for those with severe Shen disharmonies.

Following are some suggested routines.

Gentle Swaying   This encourages flexibility physically and psychologically. Practice this exercise from chapter 10, page 159, for five minutes.

The Bounce   This gently massages the Organ Systems. For two to three minutes, practice this exercise from chapter 10, page 160.

Refreshing Meditation   Spend ten minutes in visualization and stretching.

Lie, sit or stand in a comfortable position.

Close your eyes halfway.

Breathe slowly and evenly, using Buddha's breath (page 157).

Imagine yourself in an environment that is soothing to you. Perhaps along the ocean or in the mountains or in your own backyard.

Allow yourself to see the colors, feel the touch of the air on your face, smell the air, feel the sun on your skin.

Now, as you exhale, feel the stress leaving your body and drifting off, out of you, out of the scene.

Feel your chest rise and fall. Imagine your stress moving up, out of your left and right foot, up slowly through your legs, hips, and belly, moving out every time you exhale. Imagine it coming from your fingertips through your arms and shoulders, out with your breath. Imagine it moving up from your neck, along the back of your head and out the top of your head with every breath.

Rest peacefully.

Breathing Cycle   Using the Buddha's breath technique explained in chapter 10 helps disperse Stagnant Liver Qi, the most common underlying pattern associated with Shen disturbance.

• Sit on the floor with legs crossed in lotus, half-lotus, or Indian style. This is important so that Qi does not enter and become stagnated in the lower body, but follows the breathing path through the torso and the head.

• Inhale to a count of four to eight, depending on what you are comfortable with. Extend your belly, filling it up from the bottom. As you inhale, turn your attention to your nose. Guide the Qi downward from your nose toward a spot in your abdomen about one to two inches below the navel. This is the dan-tien, and women should not concentrate on it during their periods. Concentrate on the solar plexus, instead.

Exhale to a count of eight to sixteen and imagine the Qi moving down the torso, around the pelvic region, and up to the tailbone.

Inhale and visualize the Qi moving up the back to the top of the shoulders.

Exhale and feel the Qi move up the back of the head and back to the nose.

One cycle may take about seventy seconds to complete. You want to set a pace that allows you to breathe comfortably and maintain concentration on the movement of Qi. Repeat five times.

Massage   Self-massage is soothing to the Shen because it stimulates and regulates the flow of Xue and Qi and provides a period of pleasure and relaxation.

Acupressure: Every day you should massage Liver 3, Pericardium 6, the Si Shen Cong—the four points on the crown of the head and Yintang, between the eyebrows.

Probe around the point until you feel a tenderness and a slight emanation of energy. Applying a steady, even pressure, press down—don't stab—and then rock your finger gently around the point. Alternate holding the point steadily for about ten to thirty seconds, with periods of active massage.

General Head Massage: This can help ease headaches, anxiety, or depression. Follow instructions in chapter 11, page 168.

Ear massage: Focus on the Shenmen and the brain, heart, sympathetic, and liver points. See pages 178–184 for the location of the points.

Reflexology: Use the head, brain, and adrenal points on your foot and hand. See pages 191–193 for the location of the points.

In addition, receiving a professional massage once a week will provide the kind of thorough Shen relaxation and Qi stimulation that is difficult to do for yourself. You should choose the style of massage that is most soothing to you.

Soaks   Soaks and compresses are effective in calming the Shen because they can help move the Qi and offer a spirit-lifting time of self-indulgent pleasure.

Sleep-Ease (page 194), a chamomile-valerian soak, is highly recommended.

Nutritional Supplements   Herbs are more effective in treating disturbed Shen than supplements. However, there are several that, when combined with the other elements of the comprehensive program, can offer support for the Shen. Phosphatydl choline, lecithin, calcium/magnesium, along with ginkgo and wheatgrass juice may decrease agitation and insomnia. Melatonin may also be used to overcome insomnia, but should not be taken for more than one to four nights. It's a hormone, and no one knows what the long-term side effects are.

STEP TWO: USING A CHINESE MEDICINE PRACTITIONER

When practical, you may want to try therapies such as acupuncture and herbs before taking Western medications for anxiety and depression, since the medications all have potentially troubling side effects. If you decide the benefits of Western medications are worth the risk (and they often are), Western medicine can be used to complement the Shen-calming powers of acupuncture and herbs.

Acupuncture

Regular acupuncture sessions targeted to address your specific diagnosis can provide relief from anxiety, panic attacks, and depression. However, since depression may indicate the presence of a serious undiagnosed illness or can be life-threatening itself, you should always see a Western doctor for evaluation.

Most Shen disturbances are associated with Liver Qi Stagnation and may also include the Heart and Kidney Failing to Communicate and the Spleen Not Feeding the Heart Xue, which may lead to Liver Fire Anxiety or Yin Deficiency Anxiety. Treatment of specific points can be determined only after an individualized diagnosis.

Six months after Jeffrey first came to the clinic, curious to find out what Chinese medicine could do for his anxiety and depression, he was able to go off Prozac. "My anxiety is finished, gone," he says. "I am much more centered, more balanced."

His initial program included a blend of Eastern and Western therapy. He was seeing a psychiatrist who prescribed the Prozac and he was receiving acupuncture—twice a week for the first month, then once a week, and now once every two weeks. He also takes herbs daily.

"I never believed it would really work," he explains. "But it did. And although Misha talks to me each time I come for a treatment to see how I am, the therapy is physical as much or more than it's verbal."

HERBAL THERAPY

Herbal therapy is generally gentler on the system than Western medications, with fewer and less serious side effects and no danger of addiction. However, when someone comes in with panic attacks or deep depression and has not been able to sleep, they may want to take a Western sleeping medication for two or three days so they can break the cycle of agitation and get some rest. Then they can go on herbs that address the underlying problems associated with Shen disturbances.

Because Shen disturbances are usually deeply rooted, it is particularly important to take herbs and Western medications only under the ongoing supervision of a doctor and/or a practitioner.

EXAMPLES OF CHINESE HERB FORMULAS FOR SHEN DISTURBANCES

Formula	Herbs in Formula	Chinese Functions	Western Diagnoses

Gui Pi Tang	Ginseng (Ren Shen)
	Astragalus (Huang Qi)
	Tang Kwei (Dang Gui)
	Longan (Long Yan Rou)
	Atractylodes (Bai Zhu)
	Saussurea (Mu Xiang)
	Poria (Fu Ling)
	Yuan Zhi (Polygala)
	Zizyphus (Suan Zao Ren)
	Baked licorice
	  (Gan Cao)
	Fresh ginger
	  (Sheng Jiang)
	Red dates (Da Zao)
		Tonifies Qi and Xue
		
		Strengthens Heart and
		  Spleen
		
		(only to be used when there
		  is no Heat)
			Insomnia
			Functional uterine bleeding
			Aplastic anemia
			Palpitations

Shen Gem™	Ginseng (Ren Shen) Poria (Fu Ling) Atractylodes (Bai Zhu) Zizyphus (Suan Zao Ren) Astragalus (Huang Qi)	Vitalizes Heart Xue Tonifies Spleen, Heart, Qi, and Xue Calms Shen	Insomnia Memory loss Palpitations

Formula	Herbs in Formula	Chinese Functions	Western Diagnoses
	Tang Kwei (Dang Gui) Salvia (Dan Shen) Amber (Hu Po) Yuan Zhi (Polygala) Longan (Long Yan Rou) Saussurea (Mu Xiang) Dried ginger (Gan Jiang) Licorice (Gan Cao) Cardamom (Sha Ren)	(only to be used when there is no Heat)	
Ease Plus™	Oyster shell calcium (Mu Li and Long Gu) Bupleurum (Chai Hu) Ginseng (Gan Jiang) Pinellia (Ban Xia) Scutellaria (Huang Qin) Cinnamon (Gui Zhi) Rhubarb (Da Huang) Saussurea (Mu Xiang)	Invigorates Liver Qi Sedates Liver Yang Tonifies Spleen Qi Calms Shen	Drug and alcohol withdrawal symptoms Insomnia Stress disorders Migraines Gastric ulcers
Bupleurum and Dragon Bone	Bupleurum Poria Pinellia Rhubarb Cinnamon Scutellaria Red dates Ginseng Ginger Oyster shell Dragon bone	Purges Heat Dispels Dampness Purges Intestines Calms Shen	Drug and alcohol withdrawal symptoms Epilepsy Hypertension
Schizandra Dreams™	Kava Kava (piper methysticum) Schizandra (Wu Wei Zi) Calcium carbonate from Oyster shell (Mu Li), Dragon bone (Long Gu), and Amber (Hu Po)	Nourishes the Heart Calms the Shen	Insomnia Gastric ulcers Anxiety attacks
Cerebral Tonic	Angelica sinensis (Dang Gui) Zizyphus (Suan Zao Ren) Cistanche (Rou Cong Rong) S. Biota (Bai Zi Ren)	Tonifies Xue, Heart, and Kidney Nourishes the brain Calms Shen	Insomnia Palpitations vPanic attacks Anxiety Headaches

Formula	Herbs in Formula	Chinese Functions	Western Diagnoses
	Gastrodia (Tian Ma) Polygala (Yuan Zhi) Walnut kernels (Hu Tao Ren) Arisamatis (Tian Nan Xing) Acorus (Chang Pu) Lycium fruit (Gou Qi Zi) Succinum (Hu Po) Dens Draconis (Long Chi) Schizandra (Wu Wei Zi)		
Aspiration™	Polygala (Yuan Zhi) Vervain (Herba verbena) Gambir (Gou Teng) Gardenia (Zhi Zi) Albizzia flowers (He Huan Hua) Damiana (folium turnerae aphrodisiaciae) Peony (Bai Shao) Tang-Kwei (Dang Gui) Pinellia (Ban Xia) Poria (Fu Ling) Aquilaria (Chen Xiang) *A combination of Chinese and Western herbs*	Clears Stagnant Liver, Qi, and Xue Resolves Dampness Clears Heat Resolves Food Stagnation and phlegm	Depression Epigastric pain Constipation
Calm Spirit™	Taurine Magnesium aspartate Enzymes: Peroxidase, catalase, amylase, protease, and lipase Herbs: Biota (Bai Zi Ren) Tang-Kwei (Dang Gui) Fu Shen (Fu Shen) Polygala (Yuan Zhi) Zizyphus (Suan Zao Ren) Peony (Bai Shao) Ophiogon (Mai Men Dong)	Calms Shen Nourishes Xue and Heart Yin Moistens the Intestines	Depression Anxiety Insomnia Constipation

Formula	Herbs in Formula	Chinese Functions	Western Diagnoses
	Codonopsis (Dang Shen) Succinum (Hu Po) This formula blends Eastern herbs and Western supplements		
Xiao Yao San (ease powder)	Bupleurum (Chai hu) Angelica sinensis (Dang Gui) White peony (Bai Shao) Atractylodes (Bai Zhu) Poria (Fu Ling) Peppermint (Bo He) Fresh ginger (Sheng Jiang) Baked licorice (Gan Cao)	Harmonizes Liver and Spleen functions Regulates Liver Xue Tonifies Xue	Mild depression Chronic hepatitis Functional uterine bleeding PMS
Woman's Balance™	Bupleurum (Chai Hu) Tang-kwei (Dang Gui) White peony (Bai Shao) Salvia (Dan Shen) Poria (Fu Ling) Atractylodes (Bai Zhu) Cyperus (Xiang Fu) Citrus (Chen Pi) Moutan (MuDan Pi) Gardenia (Zhi Zi) Dried ginger (Gan Jiang) Licorice (Gan Cao)	Invigorates congested Liver Qi Nourishes Liver Xue and Yin Strengthens Spleen Qi Harmonizes Liver and Spleen	Mild depression PMS Hepatitis Headaches

STEP THREE: GOING TO A WESTERN DOCTOR

Depression, panic attacks, anxiety and stress-related disorders can benefit enormously from Western intervention, particularly if used in conjunction with Chinese medicine. Chinese therapy can often ease the negative impact of the Western medication without interfering with positive therapy.

The reason to use Western drugs to treat what the West identifies psychological disorders is twofold. First, in the past ten years, there has been a revolutionary change in Western medicine's understanding of the role of body chemistry in neuropsychological problems such as depression and obsessive-compulsive disorder. This has led to the development of medications that help compensate for deficiencies and produce changes in the underlying chemistry of the body. That in turn eases the symptoms of the disharmony. Western medicine is actually getting closer to the Chinese viewpoint in these areas. Second, some Western syndromes that are related to Shen disturbance, such as depression, may be life-threatening if not ameliorated immediately. Often, Western intervention can remove the short-term threat.

Your Western baseline should include a physical work-up to eliminate the presence of a serious underlying disease; evaluation to determine possible physical origins of the disorder; and a complete discussion of your options, including talk therapy and medications, with an in-depth discussion of their benefits and side effects.

STEP FOUR: OTHER HEALERS

Psychotherapy, spiritual healers, body work practitioners, self-help and support groups and twelve-step programs are tremendously important in any program to restore harmony to the Shen. Chinese medicine recognizes the positive influence of functioning as a member of a group. The balance of Yin/Yang that joins the mind/body/spirit also connects each person to the world at large and to each individual in it. When that connection is reinforced and strengthened by positive interdependence, the internal harmony of the mind/body/spirit is also strengthened.

If you decide to see an individual therapist or healer, try to arrange for her or him to talk with your Chinese medicine practitioner so they can work in concert. The therapist's diagnosis can help guide the Chinese practitioner toward targeted therapies. Also, Chinese medicine treatments may resolve some Shen problems, allowing the therapist to focus on others.

COMPREHENSIVE HEALING PROGRAM FOR CALMING THE SHEN

Self-Care	
Dietary guidelines	Eat foods that regulate or move Stagnant Qi and motivate stuck energy, those that sedate Excess Liver conditions and help ease Xue Deficiency.
	Avoid caffeine, alcohol, fatty foods, raw fruit and vegetables, excess sweets, and cold liquids or ice.
Exercise/ meditation	A daily routine: at least 20 minutes of Qi Gong exercises and 20 minutes of meditation. One half hour of aerobic activity, from walking to swimming or cycling, in addition to the Qi Gong, is recommended for those with severe Shen disharmonies.
Massage	Acupressure: Every day you should massage Liver 3, Pericardium 6, the Si Shen Cong—the four points on the crown of the head and Yintang, between the eyebrows. General head massage and ear massage Reflexology: Use the head, brain, and adrenal points on foot and hand.

Self-Care

	In addition, a professional massage once a week will provide thorough Shen relaxation and Qi stimulation.
Soaks	Sleep-Ease (page 194), a chamomile-valerian soak, is highly recommended. A ginger compress around the neck and shoulders can stimulate Stagnant Qi. (See page 197 for instructions.)
Supplements	Supplements, when combined with the other elements of the comprehensive program, can offer support for the Shen.

Using a Chinese Medicine Practitioner

Acupuncture	Treatment of specific points can be determined only after an individualized diagnosis.
Herbal therapy	There are many herb formulas that can ease Shen disharmony: some include Gui Pi Tang, Shen Gem, Ease Plus™, Bupleurum and Dragon Bone, Schizandra Dream™, Cerebral Tonic, Aspiration™, and Woman's Balance™.

Going to a Western Doctor

Obtaining a Western baseline	Your Western baseline should include a physical work-up to eliminate the presence of a serious underlying disease; evaluation to determine possible physical origins of the disorder; a complete discussion of your options, including talk therapy and medications, with an in-depth discussion of their benefits and side effects.
Other healers	Psychotherapists, spiritual healers, body work practitioners, self-help and support groups and twelve-step programs all can help restore harmony to the Shen.

CHAPTER FIFTEEN

Harmonious Cycles

A Comprehensive Program for Gynecologic Health

At one time or another, most women must contend with some unpleasant physical symptoms, such as bloating, irritability or pain, before or during their period. These are not necessarily a sign of sickness, but they do indicate that there is a degree of disharmony in the reproductive system. By following this comprehensive program, you can lessen or eliminate those unpleasant symptoms and restore harmony without resorting to over-the-counter medications or prescription drugs.

Before beginning the program, however, let's review the Chinese and Western concepts of a woman's reproductive system and the origins of disharmonies and disorders.

WOMEN'S HEALTH IN CHINESE MEDICINE

The monthly cycle depends on the harmonious functioning of the Stomach, Spleen, Liver, and Kidney Systems, and a balanced flow of Qi and Xue. Irregular periods or pain, bloating, mood swings and/or cramps are a sign that one or more of the governing Organ Systems and Qi and Xue are not in balance. It's also possible that gynecological problems have a more complex origin in a woman's emotional history, which has caused damage along the Chong Mai (or penetrating) channel.

Such emotional and physical disharmonies can produce a combination of symptoms. The Kidney controls the formation and release of the egg from the ovaries. If Kidney Qi, Yin, or Yang is weak, infertility may result. Kidney Deficiency can accompany a kind of chronic fearfulness that causes tension, irritability, or depression associated with the monthly cycle. Since Liver Qi promotes the free flow of Qi and triggers the release of Xue and the onset of the period, menstrual problems, such as cramps before or during the onset of the period and mild premenstrual headache, are usually due to Stagnant Qi. If Liver Qi is not flowing smoothly, depression and anxiety may occur in the days before the period. Excess Liver can accompany generalized anger. Conversely, anger and emotional suppression can damage Liver Qi. Stagnant Liver Qi is associated with menstrual cramps and mild headaches that subside with the onset of the period. Stagnant Liver Qi with Heat is associated with irritability, flashes of anger, a feeling of a hot sensation in the upper part of the body, and breast pain. When combined with Stomach Heat, you may experience acne, increased appetite and breast pain.

When Liver Qi Stagnation leads to Stagnant Xue, there may be Xue clots with severe headaches during the period. When Xue Stagnation is accompanied by a cold sensation, you may experience a cold sensation in the abdomen, a darker flow with dark clots and cramps that are eased by the application of warmth.

Spleen disharmony develops as either Deficient Spleen Qi or Spleen Qi Deficiency with Dampness. These syndromes are associated with digestive disturbances, sugar craving, and fluid retention. When Deficient Spleen leads to Deficient Xue, it is associated with lengthening of the cycle or missed periods and difficulty falling asleep.

THE MONTHLY CYCLE IN CHINESE MEDICINE

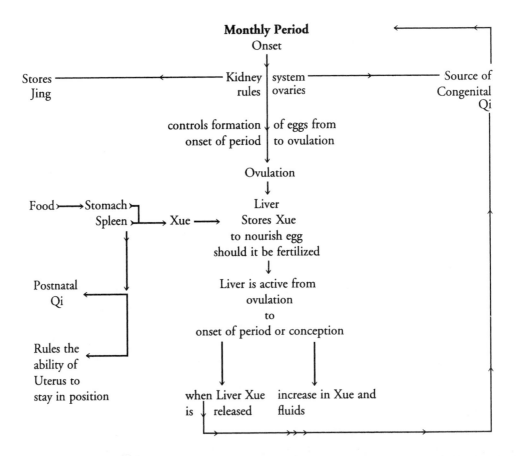

WOMEN'S HEALTH IN WESTERN MEDICINE

A woman's cycle is divided into the ovarian and the endometrial stages. The ovarian stage contains the follicular, midcycle, and luteal phases; the endometrial stage is made up of the proliferative and secretory phases. These two parts of the cycle are controlled by the interaction of various hormone-secreting organs: the hypothalamus, pituitary, and ovary. They secrete GNRH (gonadotropin-releasing hormone), gonadotropin (luteinizing hormone and follicle-stimulating hormone), and steroidal hormones (estrogen and progesterone). A normal cycle is between twenty-one and thirty-six days long. The luteal phase needs to be from twelve to fourteen days long for fertility to be robust. Menstruation itself runs one to seven days. Longer than seven days is considered abnormal. In Western medicine, disorders such as PMS and endometriosis are not entirely understood: no one is sure what

THE CHINESE CYCLE AND THE WESTERN CYCLE

The Ideal Western Cycle

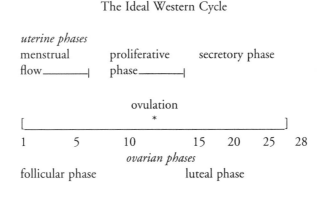

uterine phases
menstrual   proliferative   secretory phase
flow_____| phase_____|

ovulation
*
[_____]
1   5   10   15   20   25   28
                 ovarian phases
follicular phase   luteal phase

The Ideal Chinese Cycle

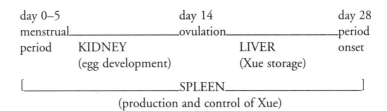

day 0–5   day 14   day 28
menstrual_____ovulation_____period
period   KIDNEY   LIVER   onset
           (egg development)   (Xue storage)
     [_____SPLEEN_____]
               (production and control of Xue)

Although this is the ideal cycle, Chinese medicine considers any regular cycle to be a healthy cycle. One woman may have a period every twenty-one days, another every thirty-five. If they are both regular, then no disharmony is indicated.

triggers either condition. When PMS is the Western diagnosis, recommendations include hormonal therapy, antiprostaglandins, and analgesics (Motrin or Anaprox), dietary changes, including avoiding caffeine, exercise, and psychotherapy. For endometriosis, the alternatives are surgery and potent but often ineffective drug therapy. Until recently, emotional components of gynecological disorders were dismissed or trivialized. Western therapies offer few targeted treatments to ameliorate emotional disturbances and associated physical complaints.

BASIC FACTS

The average age of menarche in North America is 12.5 years old. [1]

The perimenopausal stage can last two to ten years. Usually, in the beginning, there are shorter cycles (probably caused by the luteal phase becoming irregular). As menopause nears, periods are farther apart, probably because ovulation ceases. Beginning and ends of the fertility cycle are marked by long anovulatory cycles with progesterone deficiency.

The average age for menopause is fifty-one in the United States. Smokers reach menopause earlier. [2]

PART ONE: SELF-CARE FOR PREVENTION AND THERAPEUTIC TREATMENT

STEP ONE: ADOPT THE COMPREHENSIVE PROGRAM FOR STRENGTHENING ORGAN QI AND PROTECTIVE QI

A general, preventive health care routine that includes a balanced diet, regular exercise and meditation, self-massage, and other stress-reduction techniques is essential for reproductive health. That's why this gynecologic health program integrates the general comprehensive program for good health (page 203) with preventive techniques tailored to suit the unique needs of women's bodies.

For those who suffer from specific complaints, such as PMS and menopausal symptoms, there are targeted therapies.

STEP TWO: EXPAND YOUR DAILY LOG

When starting a comprehensive gynecological program, the first step is to expand your daily log from the general comprehensive program to include information on your cycle and associated physical and emotional responses. You should get in the habit of making these notations every day for at least six months, even if you stop keeping your general log after two weeks. In fact, its not a bad habit for a lifetime. If you have a well-balanced cycle, it will help alert you to the development of any disharmonies. If you are currently working to remedy an imbalance, it will alert you to triggers and help you track improvements.

The monthly log should include information on the following:

- food cravings or times when you lose your appetite for specific foods or food in general
- alcohol and caffeine consumption
- energy levels and ability to exercise
- times when sore breasts, overall heaviness or bloating, depression, or fatigue make it difficult to exercise
- Emotional ups and downs—especially times when you are irritable, cry or feel like crying, get angry or become depressed and times when your emotions are positive
- physical symptoms you suspect are associated with your cycle, such as headaches, blood sugar problems, insomnia, swollen ankles, tender breasts, swollen abdomen, cramps, acne or lower back pain
- information about the quality of your period itself: date of ovulation and feelings surrounding it; date of onset and description of quality of flow, color, texture, intensity and duration.

A review of this information over the course of several months should reveal correlations between monthly cycle, diet, exercise, emotions and physical symptoms. This information indicates how you can control or eliminate some of the troubling symptoms associated with your cycle. You'll see which times of the month you should be particularly vigilant about such things as exercising, avoiding stress and avoiding foods that exacerbate symptoms.

STEP THREE: IMPLEMENTING A GYNECOLOGICAL SELF-CARE PLAN

To keep your cycle regular, adopt a six-part plan that brings together the beneficial powers of self-care.

1. Dietary Guidelines

In addition to the diet guidelines outlined in the comprehensive program for good health, you may tailor your diet to remove Dampness and promote a balanced flow of Qi and Xue:

Eat a diet of warm, cooked foods. Be particularly careful not to eat cold, raw foods during your period, since it only increases cramping and discomfort.

Avoid excess dairy products to decrease Dampness and strengthen Spleen.

Eliminate caffeine and drink a minimum of alcohol, which increases PMS symptoms and is linked to increased breast cancer risk. Artificial stimulants of all kinds amplify gynecological disharmonies causing Liver Qi Stagnation and Liver and Heart Fire.

Eat a low-fat diet, since excess body fat increases estrogen production and can lead to various gynecological problems. A fatty diet can also increase Qi Stagnation and Dampness, which is associated with depression and lack of energy.

Increase fiber and grain in your diet to avoid premenstrual constipation.

Eliminate excess salt from your diet to ease water retention. Pure foods contribute enough salt to the diet to maintain health. The use of processed and packaged foods and the addition of salt to home-cooked meals is unnecessary and can be detrimental to your health. According to Five Phases diagnoses, excess salt injures the Kidney water, counteracts earth, and injures the Spleen.

Once a week, have a bowl of San Qi Chicken (see recipe on page 100).

Eliminate any foods that your daily log seems to have revealed as being associated with PMS, cramps, irregularity, or any of the emotional and physical symptoms surrounding the progress of your cycle. You may try reintroducing them after a one-month break by using the first-step dietary therapy program (see page 95).

2. Implementing an Exercise Plan

To regulate and move Qi and Xue so they flow smoothly, avoid excessive aerobic activities. If you're trying to reestablish a regular, symptom-free cycle, the first step is to use Yoga, Qi Gong warm-up exercises (page 159) and walking to stimulate balanced flow. Once a routine is established (daily, for 30 minutes), you can expand your exercises to include aerobics such as jogging, cycling and swimming. Exercising five times a week, forty-five minutes a day will strengthen Qi, but you should avoid exercise to the point of exhaustion or you will deplete your Qi. Your total exercise time should be about seven and a quarter hours a week, including the Yoga and/or Qi Gong and aerobics.

If you have any gynecological disharmony, weight-lifting exercises should be done only three days a week. The process of tearing down and building up muscle tissue can cause Spleen Deficiency, which could lead to a Xue Deficiency and increased menstrual problems.

3. Implementing a Meditation Plan

Stress is both a trigger and a result of gynecological problems. Meditation can alleviate the stress and diminish associated symptoms such as premenstrual depression and anxiety. Use the lotus blossom meditation (page 166) for a quick time-out from cycle-related discomfort and stress. Use the breath circulation exercise (page 163) to help ease Stagnation. Regular practice of the longer Qi meditation (page 164) can produce constitutional improvements that will do much to restore harmony.

4. *Using Self-Massage and Moxibustion for Preventive Care*

Qi Gong abdominal massage (page 171) is effective while you are having cramps and, when used regularly throughout the month, it can dispel stagnation and dampness, relieving PMS and dysmenorrhea.

Use reflexology on the hands and feet, particularly on the abdomen, womb, uterus, lower back, and brain points.

Acupressure on Liver 3 is recommended (see page 186).

Perform a monthly breast self-exam. All women over twenty should examine their breasts once a month for changes in texture, shape, color of skin and evidence of discharge from the nipples. To examine the breasts effectively, the American Cancer Society suggests you examine first one side of the breast, then the other, while lying slightly to the opposite side so that the breast is distended downward. Then lie flat on your back and repeat the examination of the center and front. Make sure you examine the area around and in your armpit as well.

In addition to the traditional Western self-exam, Western herbalist Susun Weed[3] advocates an herbal massage, done in the bath. Not only is it less intimidating a process, but it combines the monthly checkup with stress reduction. To enjoy this therapeutic soak follow these steps.

- Buy or make your own herbal oil by infusing olive or canola oil with fresh thyme, rosemary, basil, peppermint, rose petals or whatever else you like.
- Draw a warm bath.
- Pour herbal oil into the palm of your hand.
- Place both hands around one breast, thumbs pointing to the ceiling, fingers cradling the breast from underneath.
- Touch the tips of your thumbs at the top of your breast and draw them down toward the nipple.
- Repeat this motion slowly, pressing down as hard as is comfortable, but spread the thumbs apart one-half inch.
- Repeat motion until your thumbs are halfway down your breast on opposite sides.
- Add more oil at any time.
- Now, use your fingers under your breast to draw up toward the nipple. Spread them farther and farther apart until you have massaged the whole breast.

   As with the more traditional massage, if you repeat this at the same time in your cycle every month, you will become acquainted with the texture of your breasts and become alert to any variations that may require diagnostic testing by a Western doctor.

   Perform self-moxa on Spleen 6 and Ren 6 once a week for three weeks, with a week off during your period (see pages 141 and 31).

5. Using Soaks, Saunas and Compresses for Self-Healing

In general, warming compresses and brief soaks can ease some of the discomfort associated with cramps and low back pain during the onset of your period. You have to tune into what temperature is best for you. If you are already feeling too hot or dizzy, then keep the water temperature and saunas below 101° F. If you feel cold dampness, hotter compresses, soaks, and saunas can be beneficial.

Use Sleep-Ease, a chamomile-based soak to which you may also add valerian. For instructions, see page 194. Enjoy this soak for up to half an hour. You can also use ginger soaks and ginger compresses. For instructions, see the comprehensive digestive program, page 253.

6. Taking Nutritional Supplements

For all women, a daily supplement program should include essential fatty acids such as linseed oil and evening primrose oil; antioxidants, such as beta-carotene and vitamin E; one gram of vitamin C a day; calcium hydroxyapatite (from organic beef bones, if possible); chelated magnesium in a pill with calcium for balanced dosage, if possible; and a daily dose of acidophilus to protect against yeast infections and keep the digestive tract healthy.

PART TWO: ASSEMBLING THE TEAM

When it comes to gynecological health, you need to bring in Western and Eastern practitioners as part of your preventive health care plan.

WESTERN

Every woman should have a yearly Pap smear. The American Cancer Society recommends mammograms yearly over the age of fifty and at least once every two years, depending on family history, for women over forty. Screening for sexually transmitted disease is essential.

EASTERN

Chinese medicine is particularly effective for treating the powerful confluences of emotional and physical forces that influence the harmony of a woman's cycle. (For information on Chinese medicine therapies for PMS and menopausal symptoms, see the specific treatment plans that follow the general gynecologic health plan.)

STEP ONE: OBTAINING A WESTERN BASELINE

It's important to use Western screening techniques to rule out sexually transmitted diseases or cancer as the cause of any gynecological irregularities or discomfort. Western doctors may be able to offer quick therapies for some other problems as well. Even if you opt for Western treatments, take your baseline diagnosis and information on the treatment to a Chinese practitioner. Always tell your Western doctor that you are seeking Chinese therapy, too. By seeing a Chinese doctor, you can receive treatment that will ease any negative side effects of Western treatment and you can benefit from the balancing powers of acupuncture, herbs, and other Chinese therapies.

"At forty-six, I was diagnosed with fibroid tumors, which caused prolonged bleeding, sometimes for a month at a time," says Irene. "My gynecologist recommended that I take Provera, and we hoped to avoid surgery. My blood pressure was up to 140/90 and I was feeling pretty badly."

Irene had a hard time taking the Provera, which made her vision blurry, her moods manic, and her body bloated. She decided to try acupuncture for the bleeding.

"After a few treatments, the bleeding stopped. I went back to my gynecologist for my monthly visit and he told me that my blood pressure was also down—to 130/88. I didn't immediately see the connection. But after a few months, I could tell that it was the acupuncture treatments. They had taken care of the bleeding and my high blood pressure. Today, at fifty-three, my blood pressure is 110/70, and I have acupuncture treatments twice a month for a half hour. The treatments also kept my condition under control for five years.

"And one more thing . . . after observing my success with acupuncture, my seventy-seven-year-old mother tried it for arthritis and neck pain and has continued treatment for three years now. She drives an hour each way to receive treatments she considers 'life prolonging.' "

STEP TWO: OBTAINING A CHINESE MEDICINE DIAGNOSIS AND TREATMENT

To ascertain your gynecological health, a Chinese medicine practitioner does not do a direct examination of your reproductive organs. Rather, using the Four Examinations (see page 67), the practitioner conducts an interview to determine what disharmonies are present and to find out what symptoms are troubling you. From that, the practitioner is able to design a course that will restore harmony to your Organ Systems and Essential Substances and, as a consequence, alleviate your gynecological problems.

Acupuncture and Moxibustion

Qi and Xue harmonizing treatments once a month will promote gynecological harmony. They are effective in influencing the Spleen, Liver, and Kidney Systems at appropriate stages of the cycle to preserve or restore regularity and harmony.

Acupuncture can also be used in a general way to impact the channels that are particularly important in maintaining a harmonious reproductive cycle. The four extraordinary channels that govern the cycle are: the Chong, Dai Mai, Ren Mai (the conception channel) and the Du Mai (the governing channel).

The Ren Mai is related to all the Yin Organs and channels and in charge of transporting of the Jing, Xue and body fluids. As conduit of Xue, which is a Yin substance, the Ren Mai plays a large part in the woman's cycle. It also supports Qi, Xue and body fluids for supply to the fetus. If the Ren Mai is weak, women may miss periods, become infertile, or have difficulty with pregnancy or labor. The Du Mai is the master of all Yang energy and, with the Ren Mai, it regulates the balance of Yin/Yang, which in turn regulates Qi and Xue and keeps the functions of the uterus normal. The lack of Yang due to a Du Mai disturbance might lead to spotting accompanied by vaginal discharge. One other channel that is important, the Dai Mai or belt channel, is closely associated with the Liver and Gallbladder. If the Liver is not moving Qi correctly, it cannot absorb female hormones as it should. Headaches associated with the menstrual period may occur.

Moxibustion For general gynecological health, maintenance centers on Ren 6 (page 31) and Spleen 6 (page 141) plus back points along the Urinary Bladder (UB 20 and 23) and the sacrum or lower back (page 142).

Herbal Treatments

Most herbal formulas are designed to treat specific disharmonies and are not appropriate for preventive care. However, there are some herbal soups that can help regulate the flow of Qi and Xue and as such offer general herbal support for gynecological health. (For herbal treatments for specific gynecologic complaints, see the sections below on PMS and menopausal and premenopausal symptoms.)

HERBS FOR GENERAL GYNECOLOGICAL HARMONY

Herb Soup	Herbal Content	Chinese Therapeutic Effect
Dang Gui Chicken Soup (recipe on page 99)	Dang Gui (angelica sinensis)	Eat once a week to strengthen Spleen and Xue
San Qi Chicken (recipe on page 100)	San Qi (pseudoginseng)	Eat once a week to strengthen and circulate Xue

STEP THREE: BRINGING IN OTHER MODALITIES

Your treatment plan can be expanded in several ways. To increase Shen harmony and to reduce irritability, mood swings, stress and/or depression, you may want to include other forms of Eastern meditations, biofeedback, hypnosis, or psychotherapy. To alleviate digestive problems associated with your cycle, you may want to try an Ayurvedic diet that dispels the imbalance. Japanese abdominal massage can also ease digestive problems and alleviate pain associated with your period. (See the reference section for sources of information on instruction and practice.)

FREEING THE QI: THE COMPREHENSIVE PROGRAM FOR PMS MANAGEMENT

To ease PMS symptoms, you want to expand the general gynecologic program to include targeted therapies.

PMS is a loose collection of symptoms triggered by hormonal shifts that afflict an estimated 80 percent of all women during the last week or two of their menstrual cycle. The symptoms include increased appetite and sugar cravings, fatigue, headaches, dizziness, palpitations, depression, weight gain, breast tenderness, emotional volatility, vaginal infections, constipation, worsening of allergies and acne or skin eruptions. For 10 to 20 percent of women, the syndrome is incapacitating.

In Chinese medicine, these symptoms are associated with various disharmonies: Stagnant Liver Qi, Depressive Liver Fire, Deficient Heart Xue/Deficient Liver Xue, Stomach Heat and Deficient Spleen Qi with Dampness.

To eliminate these often debilitating symptoms and restore harmony to the Organ Systems, Essential Substances, and channels, follow the general comprehensive program for gynecologic health (page 236), plus the following steps.

STEP ONE: ADDITIONAL DIETARY GUIDELINES

In addition to the general gynecologic guidelines, women with PMS should eliminate all refined sugars from the diet; eliminate decaffeinated coffee, chocolate, and dark sodas; reduce the fat content of their diet to 25 percent of daily calories; avoid over-the-counter diuretics and instead, adjust the diet to eliminate excess salt and increase grains and fiber; and drink 48 ounces of filtered water or spring water a day.

STEP TWO: NUTRITIONAL SUPPLEMENTS

No nutritional supplements should be taken without talking to your Western doctor and/or Chinese practitioner since there may be contraindications you don't know about.

Vitamin B_6 may provide some relief in doses between 250 and 500 mg a day. The proof that it works is anecdotal at this point.

Science News reports that women with PMS have lower zinc levels during the luteal phase—that is, between ovulation and onset—and zinc deficiency may be associated with PMS symptoms. However, only take zinc supplements under the direction of your practitioner. Minimal amounts of zinc are needed as supplements, and there have been reported side effects from doses as small as the RDA of 15 mg a day. Side effects include interference with copper and iron metabolism leading to a negative impact on serum lipids (fat in the blood) and immune function.[4]

Calcium hydroxyapatite and magnesium supplements should be considered. Chocolate cravings associated with PMS may in fact result from magnesium deficiency, since chocolate is relatively high in magnesium. Calcium is important for general gynecologic health plus as a preventive measure against osteoporosis, the brittle bone syndrome that afflicts so many women after menopause.

STEP THREE: ADDITIONAL HERBAL TREATMENTS

There are several Chinese herbal formulas that are designed to treat disharmonies associated with symptoms of PMS. Do not self-medicate. A licensed practitioner should do a thorough diagnostic examination and then prescribe appropriate herb therapy. Your practitioner may recommend the following formulas, depending on your diagnosis.

STEP FOUR: BRINGING IN ADDITIONAL MODALITIES

One of the most innovative solutions to PMS is the use of natural progesterone cream to provide a small boost in the level of natural progesterone in the later half of the cycle.

The common theory about PMS is that it stems from elevated levels of estrogen. Another view holds that it is the relative lack of progesterone in relation to the amount of estrogen that causes PMS. Western science does prescribe synthetic progestin to counter menopausal symptoms, but this chemical is not a satisfactory replica of natural progesterone. In fact, progestin seems to actually inhibit the body's natural synthesis of progesterone, thereby worsening symptoms.

Wild yam and soy beans contain a chemical that can be converted into natural progesterone and is nearly identical to the molecule produced in a woman's body. By using a cream containing wild yam or soy beans along with natural progesterone, the effects of unbalanced estrogen production can often be eliminated.

WARNING

This cream should never be used without a practitioner's supervision and never in conjunction with other hormones or medicines without consulting both your Chinese and Western doctors.

CHINESE HERBAL FORMULAS TO TREAT PMS

Formula	Herbs in Formula	Chinese Functions	Western Indication
Woman's Balance™	Chai Hu (bupleurum chinense) Dang Gui (angelica sinensis) Bai Shao (paeonia lactiflora) Dan Shen (salvia miltorrhiza) Fu Ling (poria cocos) Bai Zhu (atractylodes) Xiang Fu (cyperus rotunda) Chen Pi (citrus reticulata) Mu Dan Pi (moutan radicis) Zhi Zi (Gardenia jasminoides) Gan Jiang (zingiberis oficinale, cooked) Gan Cao (glycyrrhiza)	Regulates Qi Nourishes Liver Xue and Yin Strengthen Spleen Qi Harmonizes Liver and Spleen	Menstrual disorders PMS Swollen breasts Depression Menstrual pain Irregular periods Abdominal bloating
Xiao Yao Wan	Chai Hu (bupleurum chinense) Dang Gui (angelica sinensis) Bai Shao Yao (paeonia lactiflora) Bai Zhu (atractylodes macrocephala) Fu Ling (poria cocos) Bo He (mentha) Sheng Jiang (zingiberis officinale) Gan Cao (glycyrrhiza uralensis)	Harmonizes the Liver and Spleen Regulates Liver Qi Tonifies Xue	Menstrual disorders and pain: PMS Abdominal pain Irregular periods Internal Medicine: Chronic hepatitis Pleurisy Cystic breasts
Heavenly Water™	Gotu kola (hydrocotyle asiatica) Chaste tree berries (viticis agnus-casti) Passion flower (passiflorae incarnatae) Pseudostellaria (Tai Zi Shen) Scute (Huanng Qin) Pinellia (Ban Xia) Poria (Fu Ling) Peony (Bai Shao) Tang-kuei (Dang Gui) Cyperus (Xiang Fu) Tricosanthes (Gu Lou Ren) Red dates (Da Zao) Baked licorice (Zhi Gan Cao) Citrus (Chen Pi) Blue citrus (Qing Pi)	Harmonizes: Liver Qi Stagnation Liver Fire Stomach Heat Heat Xue Deficiency Spleen Qi Deficiency Spleen Dampness	Irregular menstruation Breast tenderness Abdominal bloating Constipation Headaches Sweet cravings Acne Emotional ups and downs Depression Painful periods

SUPPORTING THE YIN: THE COMPREHENSIVE PROGRAM FOR MENOPAUSAL SYMPTOMS

To ease menopausal symptoms, you want to expand the general gynecologic program to include targeted therapies.

In Chinese medicine, the symptoms of menopause—hot flashes, palpitations, emotionality, depression, vaginal dryness, change in libido, urinary problems, and changes in skin texture—are associated with Deficient Kidney Yin, Deficient Liver Xue, Deficient Kidney Yang, and Deficient Yin and Yang of Kidney. It is important to stress that menopause is not a disease or a disorder; it is part of the natural progress of life. Any physical or emotional discomfort associated with it can be eased or eliminated.

In order to relieve your symptoms, follow the guidelines in the general gynecologic program plus the suggestions that follow here.

PART ONE: SELF-CARE

Step One: Expanding the Daily Log

Along with your daily log of your cycle, symptoms, diet, sleep patterns, exercise, stress and emotions add information about the following items.

• changes in length of cycle (shortening or lengthening) and how long your period lasts

• the quality of menstrual blood including color, heaviness of flow (light or heavy), clotting (small or large)

• how you feel during mid-cycle. Is there mid-cycle bleeding or spotting? Is there mittelschmerz (pain at mid-cycle)? What about emotional changes?

• how you feel during the week before onset of your period—is there increased depression, bloating or breast tenderness?

• any increase in skin dryness and vaginal dryness and changes in secretions

• fluctuations in your body temperature—are you hot or cold, less tolerant to changes in external temperature; do you have hot flashes, night sweats?

Step Two: Additional Dietary Guidelines

Some foods contain phytoestrogen, which can help ease the symptoms of menopause caused by lack of estrogen. In some societies, half the dietary intake contains foods that have phytoestrogens, but in the United States, less than 10 percent of our food comes from such sources. Estrogen-containing foods that have been researched and found to raise blood levels of estrogen are soy flour, linseed oil, and red clover sprouts. [5]

Foods high in calcium and magnesium are recommended as well, although dairy products are generally discouraged. Dietary fat should be kept low, especially during perimenopause, when estrogen levels are unopposed by progesterone.

Step Three: Additional Exercise Guidelines

Weight-bearing exercise is an important part of any perimenopausal or menopausal program. It is associated with increased calcium uptake and increased bone density. It's important to work both the lower and upper body. Doing weight-bearing exercises on only one part of the skeleton will not spread the benefit throughout the body. Again, however, you should only pump iron three times a week to avoid damaging the strength of Spleen and thus cause a Xue Deficiency.

Aerobic exercise is recommended for those who find they gain weight through menopause or who are at risk for heart disease. Remember, heart disease is the major killer of women over fifty.

Step Four: More Soaks and Compresses

For hot flashes, cooling soaks in peppermint or chamomile are recommended (see page 195).

Step Five: Additional Self-Massage

Ear Massage   For general menopausal symptoms, try additional ear massage every day using the uterus point, the endocrine point, the ovaries point, the sympathetic point, the Shenmen point, and the Kidney point (see page 179).

Acupressure   Rub the following points once a day for about ten minutes: Spleen 6, Kidney 3 and Stomach 36. For hot flashes, massage Heart 6, Kidney 7, Liver 2, and Kidney 6. (See pages 140–144 and 186 for the location of these points.)

Moxibustion   If you are having hot flashes, moxa should not be used without first consulting a practitioner, but it can be soothing for problems of fatigue and vaginal dryness. Use Stomach 36, Spleen 6 and Ren 6.

PART TWO: ASSEMBLING THE TEAM

When it comes time to bring in a Western doctor, Chinese practitioner, and others who offer health care and healing, you want to remember these facts.

Menopause is not a disease. Avoid practitioners who treat you as though it were.

Premenopausal and menopausal women should be vigilant about having regular mammograms, annual Pap smears (even after the period has stopped), and cardiovascular checkups. For women in high-risk groups (whites, fair-haired women, those who are very thin, smokers, those with a family history), a bone density scan may be recommended.

The smartest approach to menopause is to try the least harsh, most natural treatments first. That means changing your diet, increasing supplements—particularly vitamin E—reducing stress levels, increasing aerobic exercise routines, avoiding caffeine, stopping smoking—this is the single worst trigger of symptoms—and using acupuncture, herbs, massage, and meditation first.

There are a growing number of physicians who are using estrogen replacement therapy (ERT) or hormone replacement therapy (HRT) as the last resort for menopausal symptoms. Evidence is mixed about the increased risk of breast cancer among women who use ERT, although evidence that the risk of osteoporosis and heart disease is decreased appears overwhelming. However, the lifestyle changes suggested in this comprehensive program and throughout the book may also diminish the risk of brittle bones and heart disease sufficiently to make it unnecessary to use ERT.

Step One: Additional Herbal Therapy

In addition to the herbal soups outlined in the general gynecologic program, your Chinese medicine practitioner may suggest that you take the following herbal formulas.

HERBAL FORMULAS TO TREAT MENOPAUSE

Formula	Herbs in Formula	Chinese Function	Western Diagnosis
Two Immortals™	Wu Wei Zi (schizandra) Mu Li (oyster shell) Yin Yang Huo (epimedium) Ba Ji Tian (morinda) Dang Gui (angelica sinensis) Nu Zhen Zi (ligustrum) Han Lian Cao (eclipta) Damiana (folium turnerae aphrodisiacae) Gotu Kola (radix hydrocotyle asiaticae) Tai Zi Shen (pseudostellaria) Da Zao (red dates) Zhi Mu (anemarrhena) Huang Bai (phellodendron) Zhi Gan Cao (baked licorice) Xuan Shen (scrophularia) Ba Yue Zhu (eight moon fruit)	Tonifies Liver Blood Nourishes Kidney Yin Tonifies Kidney Yang Tonifies Heart Blood Tonifies Spleen Qi	Menopause Symptoms: Hot flashes Night sweats Depression Uterine bleeding Irritability
Zhi Bai Di Huang Wan	Shu Di Huang (rehmannia) Shan Zhu Yu (fr. corni) Shan Yao (dioscorea)	Moisten Yin Quell Ascending Yang	Hot flashes

Formula	Herbs in Formula	Chinese Function	Western Diagnosis
	Ze Xie (alismatis) Mu Dan Pi (moutan) Fu Ling (Poria) Huang Bai (phellodendron) Zhi Mu (anemarrhena)		
Osteoherbal™	Lu Jin (lu jin) Gui Jao (gui jao) Rou Coong Rong (cistanche) Shu Di Huang (rehmannia) Gui Ban (gui ban) Ji Xue Tang (milletia) Zou Ma Tai (ardesia) Gui Zhi (cinnamon twig) Chuan Xiong (ligusticum) Chi Shao (red peony) Mu Gua (chaenomelis) Wu Zhu Yu (evodia) Dang Shen (codonopsis) Dang Gui (tang kwei) Gan Cao (licorice)	Strengthens bones Invigorates the Xue Tonifies Organ Qi Tonifies Yang	Easy bone fractures Weak back and limbs
Zuo Gui Wan	Cooked rehmannia Discorea Lycium Fructus corni Cuscita Cyathula Deer antler Tortoiseshell	Replenish the Liver and Kidney Yin	Dizziness Night sweats Sensation of heat in hands and feet Infertility Amenorrhea Uterine bleeding
Er Zhi Wan	Ligustrum Eclipta	Tonify Liver and Kidney	Weakness and soreness in lower back Dream-disturbed sleep Dry mouth and throat Premature graying

Step Two: Acupuncture and Moxibustion

Treatment is individualized to suit changing symptoms over the course of the premenopausal and menopausal interval. Whenever you receive treatment, you need to make a commitment of at least three months. If you go once a week and your practitioner is adept, you should see a dramatic change by your fourth cycle.

Step Three: Additional Supplements

For information on the use of natural progesterone cream to ease the symptoms of menopause, see the PMS section above.

Harmonious Cycles: A Comprehensive Program for Gynecologic Health

General Self-Care	
Self-monitoring	Keep a daily log of diet, emotions, physical symptoms, and energy levels along with a record of your cycle: when you ovulate, when you have abdominal pain or distention, when your period starts, its duration, and a description of its quality—heavy, scanty, clotty, etc. Over time, try to correlate physical and emotional symptoms with pace of cycle and your diet, stress levels, exercise routines, sleep patterns, etc.
Diet	Eat a diet of warm, cooked, low-fat foods. Increase fiber and grain to avoid premenstrual constipation. Avoid excess dairy products, eliminate caffeine and excess salt, and drink a minimum of alcohol. Eliminate any foods that your daily log seems to have revealed as being associated with PMS, cramps, irregularity or any of the emotional and physical symptoms surrounding the progress of your cycle.
Moxibustion	Ren 6 and Spleen 6 are particularly good for self-moxa.
Massage	Qi Gong abdominal massage for cramps and to dispel Stagnant Qi and Xue; ear massage, reflexology and acu-massage on Liver 3 is recommended. A monthly breast massage and self-exam is important for all women.
Exercise	Qi Gong and or Yoga, daily for 30 minutes. Once that routine is established, add aerobics such as jogging, cycling and swimming, no more than 5 times a week, 45 minutes a day.
Meditation	Use the Lotus Blossom (page 166) and the Central Qi Meditation (page 164) to ease stress.
Nutritional supplements	Essential fatty acids in linseed oil and evening primrose oil Antioxidants: vitamin E and beta-carotene Vitamin C Calcium hydroxyapatite and magnesium Acidophilus to protect against yeast infections
Compresses and Soaks	Ginger compresses and soaks and lukewarm chamomile baths

PMS Self-Care (The general guidelines above plus . . .)	
Dietary guidelines	In addition to the general dietary guidelines given above, women with PMS should: eliminate all refined sugars from the diet; eliminate decaffeinated coffee, chocolate, and dark sodas; reduce fat content of diet to 25 percent of daily calories; and avoid

	over-the-counter diuretics. Adjust diet to eliminate excess salt, increase grains and fiber. Drink 48 ounces of filtered water or springwater a day.
Nutritional supplements	In addition to supplements suggested in the general women's program, the chapter provides details of other supplements that may ease symptoms.

Menopausal Symptoms Self-Care (See general guidelines above, plus . . .)	
Self-monitoring	Along with your daily log of your cycle, symptoms, diet, sleep patterns, exercise, stress, and emotions, record information about changes in length of cycle (shortening or lengthening); how long your period lasts; quality of menstrual blood including color, heaviness of flow (light or heavy), clotting (small or large). Is there mid-cycle bleeding or spotting? What about emotional changes or PMS? Note increase in skin dryness and vaginal dryness and changes in secretions. Note fluctuations in temperature: Hot flashes? Night sweats?
Additional dietary guidelines	Some foods contain phytoestrogens, which can help ease the symptoms of menopause caused by lack of estrogen.
Additional exercise recommendations	Weight-bearing exercise 3 times a week; aerobic exercise as frequently as feels good.
Soaks	For hot flashes, cooling soaks in peppermint or chamomile are recommended.
Self-massage	Ear massage: daily. Acupressure: daily for ten minutes.
Moxibustion	Moxa should not be used if you are having hot flashes without first consulting your practitioner, but it can be soothing for problems of fatigue and vaginal dryness.

The General Program: Adding Practitioners to the Healing Team	
Obtaining a Western Baseline	For screening for cancers and sexually transmitted diseases, see a gynecologist yearly.
Chinese Medicine Evaluation and diagnosis	Using the four examinations, the practitioner will survey your general health and identify any problems that might cause disharmony in the reproductive organs.
Acupuncture	Monthly treatments on four extraordinary channels (Du Mai, Ren Mai, Chong Mai and Dai Mai) maintains harmony of the reproductive organs.

The General Program: Adding Practitioners to the Healing Team	
Moxa	In addition to the points you can do at home, a practitioner may do those on your back, such as Urinary Bladder 20 and 23 and on the lower back.
Herbs	Dang Gui Chicken Soup and San Qi Chicken Soup eaten once a week dispel dampness and keep Xue flowing smoothly.
Other therapies	To reduce irritability, mood swings, stress and/or depression, include other forms of Eastern meditations, biofeedback, hypnosis or psychotherapy. To alleviate digestive problems associated with the cycle, you may want to try an Ayurvedic diet and Japanese abdominal massage (see the reference section for sources of information on instruction and practice).

The PMS Program: Adding Practitioners	
Herbal therapy	Woman's Balance™, Xiao Yao Wan and Heavenly Water™ are three formulas that alleviate the symptoms of PMS. Use only under the supervision of a trained practitioner.
Additional modalities	One of the most innovative solutions to PMS is the use of natural progesterone cream to provide a small boost in the level of natural progesterone in the latter half of the cycle. Warning: This cream should never be used without a practitioner's supervision and never in conjunction with other hormones or medicines without consulting both your Chinese and Western doctors.

Menopausal Symptoms: Adding Practitioners	
Herbal therapy	Zhi Bai Di Huang Wan, Osteoherbal™, and Two Immortals™ are effective in easing hot flashes, mood swings, urinary problems, depression and weak bones.
Acupuncture and moxibustion	Treatment is individualized and changes over time as symptoms of menopause change.
Additional modalities	Natural progesterone (not progestin) eases estrogen-related symptoms without estrogen replacement therapy. Not to be used without supervision of a practitioner or in conjunction with other medications or hormones.

CHAPTER SIXTEEN

Supporting the Center

Digestive Disorders Management Program

For thousands of years, Chinese medicine doctors have had a profound under-standing of how important a nutritious diet and good digestion are in preventing disharmony in the mind/body/spirit. Recently, Western science has made break-throughs in research confirming, in Western terms, exactly how powerful diet is in preventing and/or causing a whole range of illnesses from colon and breast cancer[1] to allergies and irritable bowel syndrome. Yet millions of us suffer daily digestive upset and chronic digestive illnesses. Antacids, laxatives, and millions of other over-the-counter stomach remedies are downed in a futile attempt to make our bellies feel better. Millions of dollars' worth of prescription drugs, from steroids to Tagamet, are taken to ease problems that stubbornly resist available Western treatments.

Whether you have a chronic digestive disorder or an acute attack, this compre-hensive program offers a way to use self-care and assemble a team of practitioners to support your healing efforts.

PART ONE: A SIX-STEP SELF-CARE PLAN FOR PREVENTION AND THERAPEUTIC TREATMENT

Step One: Daily Log

When starting a comprehensive digestive program, the first step is to keep a log for a week or two, paying special attention to diet in relationship to daily activities, sleep patterns and your physical and emotional responses throughout the day. Over time, possible correlations between diet, emotion and symptoms of digestive prob-lems should emerge. These will then give you clues as to wise self-care and will help your practitioner(s) prescribe effective treatment. (For information on how to establish and interpret your log, see chapter 13, page 203.)

Your Diet When considering your diet in relation to digestive disorders, note in your log those foods that obviously make you feel sleepy, tired or gassy; those that increase nervousness, change stools, trigger sneezing or congestion within an hour of eating, or those that cause stomach or intestinal pain.

Your Emotions   When considering diet in relation to emotions, compare your log of times when you eat certain foods with the log of times when you notice an increase in worry, agitation or tension. Also write down if becoming emotional causes pain or tension in the area beneath your breastbone. Note if you become more gassy when you eat while you are upset or if your appetite increases or decreases with a particular emotion.

Overall Energy Levels   Track the daily ebb and flow of your energy. Do you have morning grogginess? An afternoon slump? Do you get tired after eating certain foods or eating in general? What time of day is your energy at the lowest? Compare your findings with your log for diet and emotions. Can you see a pattern between low energy, eating certain foods and experiencing certain emotions?

Physical Symptoms   Make a note of your general aches and pains; cravings for sugar, chocolate, or caffeine; stiff joints, headaches, stuffy or runny nose, itchy eyes, grumbly, gassy or upset stomach, etc. Again you want to see if there is a relationship between emotions, diet and physical symptoms.

Step Two: Implementing a Diet Program

For preventive self-care, it's a good idea to increase your intake of grains, legumes and vegetables. You also should cut down on red meats and fats, and follow a varied diet that includes many foods. (See the dietary guidelines in chapter 13 for more information.)

For self-care treatment of digestive disorders, it is vital to eat a diet of cooked, warm foods and to avoid raw, uncooked foods of any kind. That will help strengthen the Spleen/Stomach, which are generally weak when digestive disharmony occurs.

In addition, eat as simply as possible to give your body time to heal. Do not over-eat or skip any meals. Too much or too little food can create additional digestive problems.

Generally, you should have your largest meal at midday. Eating large meals in the evening or eating before going to bed puts a strain on the Spleen and Stomach Systems. If you already have a weakened Spleen, however, you may find that you feel best if you eat small meals frequently throughout the day.

Follow the First-Step Dietary Therapy Program (page 95) to break the cycle of digestive upset.

Identify those foods that you suspect may aggravate the condition by evaluating your self-monitoring log. Eliminate those foods from your diet. After four days, introduce one back into your diet. Observe the results. If all goes well, you may continue eating that food, but no more than once every four days. You may introduce each eliminated food back into your diet on a four-day rotation. If any one produces a symptomatic reaction, it should be taken out of your diet, at least for the next several months.

Take *Lactobacillus acidophilus* for both prevention and treatment of digestive upset and parasites. Yogurt doesn't pack enough live cultures into one serving to provide as much help as the pill or powder form. (See page 113 for additional information.)

Step Three: Implementing an Exercise/Meditation Plan

The methods of exercise you'll choose to help digestive disharmony depend on your Chinese diagnosis. If the Qi is weak and you experience fatigue, lack of appetite and a feeling of fullness after eating very little, then try mild Qi Gong exercises, such as numbers one and two on pages 159–160 and the breathing exercises on page 163. Done three to four times a week, they will help strengthen the Qi and ease the symptoms.

If Qi stagnation is the diagnosis (symptoms include gas, irritability and bloating), the digestive disorder will respond to more vigorous exercise five to seven days a week. Recommended exercises such as jogging, cycling, fast walking, and other aerobics should not be done to the point of exhaustion, since that can deplete instead of build Qi. Too much exercise can also deplete Xue. Women who overdo aerobic exercise may have light or no periods because of Xue Deficiency related to Qi Deficiency.

Weight lifting on machines or using free weights should only be done every other day, since the process of tearing down the muscles to build them up can cause a Spleen Deficiency, which would worsen any digestive problems.

You can, however, engage in Yoga, Qi Gong exercises (see page 159) and Tai Chi without worry about detrimental effects.

Step Four: Using Compresses and Soaks for Digestive Problems

In general, warming compresses and brief soaks ease some of the discomfort of digestive disorders; however, don't use them after eating. If you are feeling weak, use warm, not hot, water.

Use ginger compresses to warm and tonify the abdominal area. To make a ginger compress, grate a third of a large ginger root. Place the grated ginger in an unbleached square of cheesecloth and tie it securely. Place in one to two quarts of boiling water for ten minutes. Remove the bag of ginger from the water and set it aside. Take one cup of tea from the pot. Add one-half to one teaspoon dried ginger before drinking. Soak a washcloth in the remaining ginger brew in the pot. Wring it out. Apply it to your abdomen. Repeat applications until you feel very warm and comfortable. Drink the ginger tea.

Other compress alternatives include Hydrocollator packs that you heat in a boiling pot of water and microwaveable herbal heat packs (usually made with yucca, a Southwestern cactus) that become damp when heated.

For a soak, draw a chamomile or chamomile-valerian bath, using the recipe for Sleep-Ease on page 194.

Step Five: Using Massage for Self-Healing

Many massage techniques can ease discomfort and restore balance in digestive disorders.

Self-acupressure can ease the discomfort of digestive disorders. Concentrate on Stomach 36 and Spleen 6 (for stomach pain). See the diagram on pages 186 and 141 for location of points. Follow the acupressure techniques described for these points on page 173. Repeat at least once a day.

Intestinal moxibustion is a powerful self-care tool. Focus on these points for Deficiency and Cold conditions: Stomach 6, Spleen 6, Ren 6, Ren 12, and Stomach 25. Du 20 strengthens the Xue and brings up Qi. It is particularly effective for Qi Deficiency diarrhea and organ prolapse. Almost anyone can moxa Stomach 36 for Qi tonification unless he or she has a high fever or huge amounts of excess energy. Don't moxa when there is a sign of Heat problems (fever, bloody stools, or burning diarrhea) without a practitioner's prescription. See pages 31, 141 and 186 for a diagram of these points.

Try ear massage. The illustration of the ear with the points for massage (ear-Shenmen, ear-Stomach, ear-Spleen, ear-Large Intestines) can be found on page 179. Follow the massage techniques for these points, which are explained on page 173.

Use reflexology. See the illustration of the foot with points highlighted on page 193.

Hara massage, a Japanese abdominal massage, is especially soothing to those with digestive disorders.

Qi Gong abdominal self-massage instructions are on page 171.

Step Six: Nutritional Supplements

Nutritional supplements may be difficult for a person with severe digestive disorders to absorb. That's why the program begins with dietary changes, acupuncture, mild herbal formulas and exercise. Once digestive stability has been established, supplements can be added, although several of them require the supervision of a doctor or practitioner. General recommendations include:
- a low dose of B-complex with minerals
- vitamin C to bowel tolerance (When you get gas or loose stools, reduce the dosage slightly and continue at that level. If you have ongoing diarrhea, do not take.)
- Psyllium seed and husk (found in every pharmacy and health food store). This helps both diarrhea and constipation. Purchase products without added sugar. If

your digestive program includes Chinese herbs (particularly in pill form), the dosage of psyllium may be lowered because of the high fiber content of the herbs.

• Chromium picolinate (GTS), which reduces cholesterol and promotes lean body mass, also helps ease food cravings, particularly for sugar, caffeine and chocolate. Take two 50 mcg pills immediately after the meal that precedes the time of day you usually experience the craving. For example, if you have the food craving in the afternoon, then take the chromium after lunch. If the craving occurs primarily at night, take the pills after dinner. Some people may need to take it two or three times a day. [2]

• Lactase pills, for lactose intolerance, can help when it's difficult to avoid all dairy products. (Best results are from lactase pills without other additives such as sugar.) Better yet, avoid dairy altogether, since dairy products tend to promote dampness. People with chronic digestive problems tend to have Deficient Spleen and be damp. Eating dairy puts a stress on the digestive system.

• Additional forms of acidophilus may be prescribed, depending on the Western diagnosis of your digestive problem. For example, if you are having trouble in your upper small intestine, then bifidus may be recommended. Depending on the strength of the acidophilus, take from one-half a teaspoon twice a day to one teaspoon three times a day or between one and three pills a day.

• Digestive enzymes are generally good for people who have trouble digesting specific types of food, who are diagnosed as having decreased hydrochloric acid, or who can't digest any meat (especially a problem for those who have been vegetarians for many years and begin to eat meat). To determine if you need digestive enzymes, consult a Western nutritionist for recommended therapy. However, many Chinese herbal formulas are enzymatic and the need for enzymes decreases or is eliminated when receiving Chinese herbal medicines from your practitioner.

• Bovine colostrum provides immune enhancement, but use it only under a practitioner's guidance.

• Citrus seed extract is appropriate for parasites and bacterial infections, but only after a Western lab evaluation indicates that the person's digestive disorder is responsive to this substance.

PART TWO: ASSEMBLING THE TEAM

Often, when people turn to Chinese medicine, they have been suffering with chronic problems that Western medicine has not been able to relieve. If you are suffering from severe gastrointestinal disorders such as Crohn's disease or irritable bowel syndrome, or if you have bloody diarrhea, expanding the treatment to include a combination of acupuncture, moxibustion, dietary changes, herbal medicine, and exercise may create the breakthrough that's needed. However, improvement doesn't usually happen overnight. Because the disharmonies that trigger these disorders are deeply rooted, it can take a full year before the problem is completely resolved. However, people with digestive disorders frequently are able to cut back on interventions such as acupuncture and herbal medicine before the year is up. They slowly return to a more normal diet. And because they have been involved in all aspects of their healing, the person knows when to return to a stricter, more therapeutic diet before the problem recurs.

Rene came into the clinic suffering from ulcerative colitis. She was afraid to go out anywhere for fear that she couldn't get to a bathroom. She was about to get fired and she was running out of hope.

"At the clinic, I was diagnosed with spleen disharmony and told I needed to bolster my immune system, change my diet, and eliminate some stress from my life. None of those things were mentioned by my Western doctors. They just said they had no idea how I got the disease or how to get rid of it.

"I was taking steroid enemas that made me gain sixteen pounds, then I had a bad reaction to the drug they gave me to compensate for the bloating. And I was taking oral medication that gave me severe headaches.

"I came for acupuncture and herbal therapy when it was clear that Western medications weren't going to help—at least not enough and not by themselves. Misha gave me Source Qi™, an herbal formula that she developed.

"I'm still on some Western medication, but now, after ten months of Chinese medicine treatments, I'm feeling much better and taking far fewer drugs. I still get acupuncture and moxibustion on my navel and legs once a week. I also get lots of other positive effects from it. If I have any other issues in my health—stress or allergies or painful periods—the acupuncture helps them, too."

Step One: Obtaining a Western Baseline

It's important to rule out cancer and other life-threatening problems or to identify an illness that can be treated quickly and effectively by Western medicine. Follow the general guidelines in the basic comprehensive program for working with a Western practitioner, and find an expert in digestive disorders who can outline your treatment options. This information and information about ongoing Western treatment should be presented to your Chinese medicine practitioner.

Step Two: Obtaining a Chinese Medicine Diagnosis and Treatment

When you go to a Chinese practitioner, it's important to establish communication between the Chinese and the Western doctors. Both practitioners should be aware of what you are doing as director of your own healing process.

At the Chinese practitioner, you can expect to be treated with herbs, acupuncture, and moxibustion.

Herbs   The following chart outlines some of the herb formulas that I've found are most effective and indicates the Chinese functions and Western diagnoses they address. Under no circumstances should you self-administer these medicines unless they are also listed in the Medicine Cabinet on page 208.

HERBAL FORMULAS FOR DIGESTIVE PROBLEMS

Formula	Herbs in Formula	Chinese Function	Western Diagnosis
Curing/Konning Pills (pill curing)	Tian Ma (gastrodia) Bai Zhi (rx. angelica) Ju Hua (chrysanthemum) Bo He (herba menthae) Ge Gen (pueraria) Tian Hua Fen (trichosanthes) Cang Zhu (atractylodes) Yi Mi (semen coix) Mu Xiang (saussurea) Hou Po (cortex magnolia) Ju Hong (pericarpium citrus) Huo Xiang (agastaches)	Regulates the Middle Burner Improves digestion Expels Wind-Cold during the summer	Food poisoning Motion sickness Gastroenteritis: viral or bacterial **Do not use if appendicitis is suspected**
Quiet Digestion™	Fu Ling (poria) Yi Yi Ren (coix) Shen Qu (shen chu) Hou Po (magnolia) Bai Zhi (angelica) Cang Zhu (red atractylodes) Mu Xiang (saussurea) Hu Xiang (pogostemon) Gu Ya (oryza) Tian Hua Fen (trichosanthes) Ju Hua (chrysanthemum) Chi Shi Zhi (halloysite) Ju Hong (citrus) Bo He (mentha) Mai Ya (malt)	Disperses Wind and Dampness Resolves Spleen Dampness Regulates the Stomach Resolves phlegm	Food poisoning Motion sickness Gastroenteritis: viral or bacterial Hangover Jet lag **Do not use if appendicitis is suspected**
Shen Ling Bai Zhu Wan	Dang Shen (codonopsis) Fu Ling (poria) Bai Zhu (white atractylodes) Jie Geng (platycodon) Shan Yao (dioscorea) Chen Pi (citrus peel) Sha Ren (amomi seed)	Strengthens Spleen Tonifies Qi Harmonizes Stomach functions Eliminates Dampness	Chronic gastroenteritis Anemia Chronic fatigue

Formula	Herbs in Formula	Chinese Function	Western Diagnosis
	Lian Zi Rou (nelumbinis seed) Bai Bian Dou (dolichoris seed) Yi Yi Ren (coix seed)		
Gui Pi Wan	Dang Shen (codonopsis) Fu Shen (sclerotium poria) Suan Zao Ren (zizyphus) Yuan Zhi (polygala) Dang Gui (angelica sinensis) Mu Xiang (saussurea) Bai Zhu (white atractylodes) Gan Cao (licorice) Long Yan Rou (longan)	Strengthens Qi Nourishes Xue Tonifies Spleen Nourishes Heart	Digestive: Abdominal pain Abdominal distention Gynecological: Irregular menstruation Leucorrhea Chronic bleeding Neurological: Insomnia Palpitations Headache
Ping Wei San	Bai Zhu (white atractylodes) Hou Po (magnolia) Chen Pi (citrus peel) Gan Cao (glycyrrhiza)	Strengthens Stomach Resolves Dampness Disperses Stagnant Qi	Gastrointestinal inflammation Flatulence Reduced digestive functions
Stomach Tabs™	Hou Po (magnolia bark) Chen Pi (citrus peel) Ban Xia (pinellia) Cang Zhu (red atractylodes) Gan Jiang (dried ginger) Gan Cao (licorice) Chai Hu (bupleurum) Gu Ya (oryza)	Disperses Stagnant Qi Resolves Spleen Dampness Dispels Food Stagnation Resolves Stomach phlegm	Flatulence Bloating Decreased intestinal permeability
Source Qi™	Chun Bai Pi (ailanthes) Huang Qi (baked astragalus) Ren Shen (white ginseng) Bal Zhu (fried white atractylodes) Fu Ling (poria) Shan Yao (dioscorea) Lian Rou (lotus seed)	Strengthens Stomach Tonifies Qi Astringes Fluids Removes Dampness	Intestinal parasites HIV diarrhea Crohn's disease Chronic shingella Intestinal bacterial infections

Formula	Herbs in Formula	Chinese Function	Western Diagnosis
	Qian Shi (euralyes)		
	Sheng Ma (cimicifuga)		
	Gan Jiang (charcoaled ginger)		
	Chai Hu (fried bupleurum)		
	Rou Dou Kou (cardamom)		
	Zhi Gan Cao (baked licorice)		
	Shen Qu (massa fermente)		
Artestatin™ **Warning: This formula is very strong and needs close supervision. Do not use with constipation.**	Qing Hao (artemesia) Shu Chi (dichroa) Bai Tou Weng (pulsatilla) Hou Po (magnolia bark) Ban Xia (pinellia) Huo Xiang (pogostemon) Bai Bian Dou (dolichos) Ren Shen (ginseng) Chen Pi (citrus) Gan Cao (licorice) Huang Lian (coptis) Cang Zhu (red atractylodes) Sha Ren (cardamom)	Expels parasites Clears Summer Heat Circulates Stagnant Qi Tonifies Spleen Tonifies Stomach	Protozoal infestations *Giardia,* Entamebiasis Amoebic dysentery Food contamination Malaria

Acupuncture and Moxibustion For severe bowel disorders such as Crohn's disease and acute irritable bowel syndrome, the recommended therapy is acupuncture and moxibustion twice a week to begin with and once a week for an extended period—from twelve to fifty-two weeks.

Moxibustion may include additional points on the Stomach and Urinary Bladder channels (ST 37; UB 25 and UB 20). See pages 141 and 142 for a diagram of the location of the points.

Step Three: Bringing in Other Modalities

The comprehensive program includes diverse therapeutic approaches, including nutritional supplements, massage, Western lab tests and medicines, psychotherapy, Ayurvedic nutritional counseling and more.

Digestive disorders often demand comprehensive treatment plans. For example, Maggie came to the clinic with severe digestive complaints after having traveled through India. I sent her for Western lab tests for bacterial infections and parasites. They found bacterial infections, systemic candidiasis and parasites.

Chinese medicine can treat yeast infections and many parasites, but I knew that unless she took antibiotics for the bacterial infection, she could not benefit from the other therapies. Even though the antibiotics were going to aggravate her yeast infection, she needed to knock out the bacterial infection first. While she took the antibiotics, our clinic provided acidophilus and treatments to tonify the Spleen and Stomach Systems, remove dampness and combat the yeast overgrowth. Once she was done with the course of antibiotics, we could treat the increased yeast infection and parasites. Over six months, her digestive system regained harmony.

If her treatment had not included both Western and Chinese methods, Maggie's therapy would not have been as effective nor her recovery as rapid.

COMPREHENSIVE HEALING PROGRAM FOR DIGESTIVE DISORDERS

Self-Care

Evaluation	Even if you are focusing on self-care, if you suffer with a digestive disorder, you should first go for a Western baseline evaluation and a Chinese medicine evaluation. You should rule out life-threatening disorders before proceding.
Self-monitoring	If your diet log reveals that you have a negative reaction to particular foods—upset stomach, gas, runny nose, headaches, cramps, anxiety, etc.—eliminate those foods for four days and reintroduce one at a time.
Diet	Follow recommended diet plan in this chapter and make sure to avoid raw foods, cold foods, and dairy, if you suffer from Dampness. Reduce caffeine and alcohol intake.
Moxibustion	Highly recommended unless there are Heat problems such as fever, bloody stools, or burning diarrhea. Then use only if prescribed by a practitioner or doctor.
Massage	Qi Gong Chinese massage, reflexology and ear acupressure are recommended.
Exercise	If the Qi is weak, Yoga and mild Qi Gong exercises; for Qi Stagnation, more vigorous exercise five to seven days a week, but don't overdo weight lifting.
Nutritional supplements	Low-dose B-complex, Acidophilus Lactase from health food store (less additives)
Compresses and soaks	If digestive disorders related to stress, use chamomile bath Ginger compresses for Cold and Deficiency Hot packs (hydrocollator for pain, cold and deficiency)
Medicine Cabinet	Curing/Konning Pills, Quiet Digestion™—herbal formulas for nausea, food poisoning, stomach flu

Adding Practitioners to the Healing Team

Chinese Medicine	
Chinese evaluation and diagnosis	Bring self-monitoring log and other evaluations, including Western baseline. Together, the practitioner(s) and client create a healing plan.
Diet	Using daily log as guide, work with practitioner to create a diet that restores harmony.
Herbs	See chart in herb chapter for examples of herbs for Spleen and Stomach patterns—additional herbs might be added for other patterns such as Stomach Heat or Liver/Gallbladder Damp Heat
Acupuncture	Points similar to or in addition to massage and moxibustion points noted above. Acupuncture would most likely be given to treat the Stomach and Spleen channels plus additional points for additional channel problems or patterns.
Moxibustion	Practitioner might recommend specific self-treatment as well as provide moxa during office treatment sessions.
Qi Gong exercise/ meditation	Practitioner may recommend that you see a Qi Gong instructor to learn routines. You should ask your instructor for specific exercises that target what's been diagnosed.
Other Therapies	Western medical doctors may prescribe medications, such as antibiotics for bacterial infections and antiparasite drugs. Other Western practitioners who may contribute to the healing process include: homeopathic doctors, psychotherapists, biofeedback specialists.
Nutritional supplements (only taken under practitioner's supervision)	Specific supplements can be targeted toward particular disharmonies. See chapter for possible recommendations for you to discuss with your doctor.
Massage	In addition to self-massage your practitioner may recommend that you try Qi Gong massage, Shiatsu, Hara massage, Swedish and other long-stroke massage; Ayurvedic hot oil massage.

CHAPTER SEVENTEEN

Movement Toward Freedom

Dependency and Addiction Detoxification Program

The potential for becoming addicted, both physically and psychologically, exists to some degree or another in most of us. Whether we succumb or not depends on an intangible mix of physical, spiritual, psychological, and circumstantial events. These days, there are few people who aren't addicted to or dependent on something: coffee, colas, chocolate, sweets, cigarettes, dieting, exercise, laxatives, marijuana, alcohol, sleeping pills, tranquilizers, cocaine in some form, heroin, uppers, downers, or the latest drug of the month. (Dependency implies a degree of physical and psychological need for the substance in order to feel good, but does not involve an actual incorporation of the substance into the patterns of your body physiology, as addiction does.)

Clearly, we live in a culture that has an addictive personality. Moderation is rarely praised. Even our attitudes toward exercise and diet turn untold thousands of people a year into addicts: addicts of not eating, overexercise, or overconcern about the body.

Addiction can create enormous health problems whether it is legal or illegal, socially acceptable or taboo. When part of the body's physiological processes are usurped by a foreign chemical substance, all kinds of imbalances can happen to everything from cell metabolism to emotions, digestion to skin tone, respiration to contemplation.

Despite this epidemic of addictions, the prognosis for society and for each person within it who has become addicted or dependent is not hopeless. Becoming free is an enormous psychological and physical challenge, but each and every person has the ability to overcome addiction, given the appropriate support and treatment.

ARE YOU ADDICTED OR DEPENDENT?

Before you turn the page and decide this program doesn't apply to you, you may want to stop and ask yourself: Am I addicted or dependent on anything? It's common to be unsure if you are or not. Many people say: "I can give up coffee any time I want." Or, "I can stop taking cocaine. I only do it for fun on the weekends." Or, "I'm not an alcoholic, I just like to unwind a little after work." They don't realize that they are fooling themselves.

If you've ever wondered if you have a problem, chances are you do. If you answer yes to any of the following points, you should seek medical help and support to unravel your dependency and restore your mind/body/spirit to balance.

1. Does your character change when you use the drug? Are you angrier? Friendlier? More at ease?
2. Is it very difficult or impossible to go for a few hours or days without the drug (even if it's just coffee) without experiencing withdrawal symptoms?
3. Have you ever changed or rearranged your life in order to keep using the drug?
4. Have you ever put yourself in a dangerous situation to get the drug?
5. Have you lost money, a job, self-esteem, or a relationship because of your addiction?
6. Have you ever lost track of hours or even a whole day while under the influence?
7. Have loved ones tried to get you to stop, but you've refused?

USING THIS COMPREHENSIVE PROGRAM

This comprehensive program offers general support to anyone trying to shake a dependency, whether it's to caffeine or cocaine. This approach has a parallel to the twelve-step model insomuch as it works for many forms of dependency and addiction. Although each addiction has its own characteristics, each shares much in common with other addictions and responds positively to the same kind of support.

In Chinese medicine, the universal principles that apply to any detox therapy are that the Shen must be calmed, the Spleen and Kidney must be supported and strengthened, and Qi must be rebalanced so it can flow harmoniously. All dietary changes, massages, exercises, acupuncture therapy, herbal remedies, psychotherapies, and other treatments are designed to rebalance the body in these ways.

That does not mean that an addiction to caffeine threatens your health as much as an addiction to heroin, but every addiction impacts the mind/body/spirit—often in ways that are unnoticed or ignored—and requires a supportive program of therapy to restore balance and harmony to the Organ Systems, Essential Substances and channels. The length of time, intensity, and particular applications of therapies should be determined by the team of health care practitioners that you assemble to help you.

COMBINING SELF-CARE WITH PROFESSIONAL HELP

Self-care is the first and the last step in overcoming addiction, but anyone seeking to break an addiction should also avail themselves of assistance from trained practitioners. The use of Western medical therapy and monitoring, Chinese medicine, support groups, twelve-step programs, individual psychotherapy and healing techniques from many other traditions is vitally important to ensure success. For most addictions, I will only treat someone who has joined a support group, twelve-step program, or is in individual therapy. It's too difficult to go through detoxification on your own. For hard drug, barbiturate or alcohol dependency, monitoring during withdrawal is important in order to avoid or respond to life-threatening physical reactions. You should never go cold turkey when getting off barbiturates, sedatives, or drugs such as Xanax, Valium and Ativan.

THE STAGES OF BREAKING FREE

As you go through this program, remember that you don't have to do everything at once. Take it one day at a time and work slowly to improve your strength and spirit. At each step, consult with your health care support team to see what is the best pace for you.

There are three stages of detoxification: acute, short-term, and long-term. In each stage, Chinese medicine is extremely effective in easing symptoms and in restoring balance to the many bodily functions that have been disrupted by the addiction.

The **acute stage** is when the physiological craving exists and physical withdrawal is in full bloom. That's when you get severe headaches during caffeine withdrawal, difficulties with speech, irritability, and anxiety during nicotine withdrawal, DT's during severe alcohol withdrawal, and hallucinations during cocaine or heroin withdrawal. Depending on the type of addiction, the reaction can last from a few days to a few months. In nicotine addiction, the acute stage lasts about three days. In heroin addiction, it can last up to a week. Methadone withdrawal may go on for several months.

The **short-term stage** is when the physical addiction is technically broken and the consequences of the physical damage become sharply felt. Psychological adjustment to the absence of the drug and the routine surrounding it can be extremely difficult. During this and the long-term stage, cravings and the feelings of physical addiction can return, making it difficult to stick to the program: "Just one cigarette to make me feel better. It's been two months. I won't go back." How many times has that been said? Almost every time, it leads to a renewal of the habit. The same is true for any substance to which you've been addicted. Once you're off the drug, there's no such thing as just a little bit.

The **long-term stage** is when all the imbalances must be faced and treated. They are physical, spiritual, and psychological. In terms of Chinese therapy, this is the stage when the emotional consequences of severe Liver imbalance must be dealt with. Many addictions are adopted in order to smother or cope with overwhelming or uncomfortable emotions. Liver Excess in the form of too much anger, too much heat, too much fear or too much depression leads to emotional suppression, which in turn damages the Liver even more and produces Liver Fire and Spleen Deficiency.

Addiction also damages the Kidney System, which is the seat of the will. In all addictions the will is compromised. Fear is also associated with the Kidney. To strengthen the will and quell fear, the Kidney functions must be rebalanced.

The ability to address the underlying causes and results of addiction are what make Chinese medicine so effective. Unlike other approaches that can do little more than mask the withdrawal symptoms, Chinese medicine actually strengthens and heals the mind/body/spirit.

BREAKING THE CAFFEINE HABIT

When you decide you want to go off caffeine, do it slowly, not cold turkey. The easiest way is to start out limiting yourself to two cups a day for three days. Then begin adding decaffeinated coffee to your high-test. On day four, brew the pot with one-quarter decaf and three quarters caffeinated coffee; on day seven, brew the coffee half caffeinated, half decaf. On day ten, make it three-fourths decaf, one fourth caffeinated. By day fourteen, switch to all decaffeinated. This avoids or minimizes withdrawal.

THE PROGRAM: BLENDING SELF-CARE WITH PROFESSIONAL SUPPORT

The key to an effective recovery program is to do at least one healing act every day. Have a massage, take a soak, practice Qi Gong, receive acupuncture treatments, practice Yoga, attend a support group or twelve-step program, or go to a psychotherapist.

STEP ONE: SELF-MONITORING

In addition to following the guidelines given for keeping a general log (see page 203), you want to expand the diary to include information on the various drugs you may use and abuse.

It's only human to ignore the extent of an addiction. That's why the daily log is so important for coming to terms with the true nature of a dependency. Record frequency and quantity of your particular dependency or addiction. Don't skip even one entry. At the end of two weeks, you'll be amazed to see how much more you partake than you realized.

For caffeine, note the quantity and time of day that you drink coffee, tea, or caffeinated colas. Although this is not often considered a serious addiction, it does have serious health implications since it is associated with irritable bowel syndrome, insomnia, fibrocystic breasts, and perhaps even aggravation of high blood pressure.

For cigarettes, give an accurate count of the number you have every day. Also note how much effort you're willing to expend to have a smoke. Will you get up from a table in a no-smoking restaurant and stand outside so you can have a smoke? Do you avoid going over to a friend's house where you know you can't smoke? Do you make late-night runs for a pack of cigarettes rather than wait until the morning because you can't survive until morning? Cigarettes aren't the only source of nicotine addiction. If you chew tobacco or smoke a pipe or cigar, log in that information as well.

For alcohol, note the time of day you drink, the kind of liquor, the location you have a drink, how much you drink, with whom you drink, and how you feel when you fall asleep and when you wake up. Note any conflict you had while drinking or about drinking. Note any time you were unable to do what you'd scheduled because you had been or were drinking. Did you miss appointments? Were you late for work? Did you break promises?

For prescription drugs, even if your doctor hasn't said anything about how much you're taking, you could still be dependent or addicted. Sleeping pills and tranquilizers are insidious pharmaceuticals and you can become dependent before you realize what's happened. If you can no longer go to sleep without taking a pill or if you hear yourself say, "I can't cope with this. I need a tranquilizer," and then take one, chances are you're in over your head. Make a note of how many pills you take and how often you need them. Also note what is going on around the time that you do take the pills. Is there particular stress or conflict? Are you angry or worried or frightened? Remember, withdrawal from barbiturates and sedatives is extremely tricky and can be dangerous, so always consult a doctor before trying to stop taking pills.

For so-called recreational and hard drugs, any use is too much as far as the health and harmony of your mind/body/spirit, but if you're ready to try a detox program, you know that already. If you're still using, keep track of your habits, how much you use the drug, how much money you spend on it, how it makes you feel, interactions and conflicts with those around you, and your physical and emotional responses.

For those of you who already have gone through withdrawal or recovery, keep track of your cravings, emotional and physical responses to withdrawal, and thoughts about staying off or going back to the drug. Make special note of positive improvements in your internal feelings and interactions with the outside world. Every day you should write out a list of the reasons you want to successfully break the addiction.

STEP TWO: OBTAINING A WESTERN BASELINE

In order to develop a complete picture of the scope of your addiction and the potentially serious repercussions on your body, you may want to have your cardiovascular system checked and to receive an HIV (AIDS) test, if appropriate, to make sure there is no neurological damage or damage to organ functions. Share your baseline with your Chinese practitioner and any other therapists you may use. Keep your Western doctor informed about the full range of treatments you are receiving.

STEP THREE: ADDITIONAL DIETARY GUIDELINES

Almost any addiction changes how people eat and affects the functioning of the digestive system. How many times have you quelled your hunger in the middle of the afternoon with a good, strong cup of coffee? Smoking is often used as a substitute for food and alcoholics and hard drug addicts are notoriously disinterested in eating. These changes in eating patterns often lead to sugar cravings and problems with low blood sugar (hypoglycemia). In addition, any chemical dependency strains the digestive system, making it sluggish and erratic. Think about what those legal drugs—coffee and cigarettes—can do to your bowels.

Help ease sugar craving and low blood sugar and rebuild the digestive system and nurture the Qi by following these suggestions.

• Try eating small meals frequently. Initially, you may do best with six small meals a day that are high in protein and complex carbohydrates. Avoid fatty meats such as beef, sausages, ribs and fried chicken. That just makes digestion more sluggish. Instead, eat broiled fish and chicken, whole grains and beans for protein that will sustain you through the day.

• Avoid all sugar, including fruits, for the initial period of withdrawal.

• Drink at least thirty-two ounces of water a day during withdrawal. Increase to forty-eight ounces in later stages.

• Increase fiber intake to offset constipation associated with withdrawal.

• Once you are through the acute and short-term stages of detox, try the cleansing diet on page 95 to set your system back in balance.

STEP FOUR: NUTRITIONAL SUPPLEMENTS

Addictions of all kinds cause depletion of vitamins and minerals in the body and put a strain on various Organ Systems and Essential Substances. A general program of nutritional support (see page 111) is essential through all stages of recovery. In addition, some recoveries benefit from targeted supplementation.

A full regime of high-potency B vitamins is vital during the early stages of detox, particularly detox from alcohol.

Detox also uncovers the full extent of immune system depletion that has happened as a result of the addiction. Those who stop smoking almost always get a sore throat, a cold, or the flu. Similar infections afflict those who are going off other drugs. To bolster immune strength, take CoQ10 (coenzyme Q10) and vitamin C to bowel tolerance. Consult your practitioner for advice on taking selenium and zinc.

Take antioxidants, beta-carotene, and vitamin E.

Calcium and magnesium taken together before sleep can help overcome insomnia during withdrawal.

STEP FIVE: EXERCISE/MEDITATION

During the acute stage, it may be difficult to do aerobic exercise, but if you can, it will release endorphins that can soothe withdrawal symptoms and help move toxins out of the body. Qi Stagnation, which is a common result of addiction, is also alleviated by aerobics. However, if your addiction has caused serious deficiencies—and it certainly can—then aerobics are only going to deplete you further.

In contrast, Qi Gong exercises, Yoga, and meditation are beneficial for everyone at any stage of withdrawal or recovery. The controlled breathing used in Eastern exercise/meditation strengthens the Kidney and harmonizes the emotions. Furthermore, the way that meditation makes thoughts flow across the mind without evoking anger or fear eases emotional suppression and helps heal the Liver. A blend of Yoga, Qi Gong and meditation, thirty to sixty minutes a day, will do a great deal to vanquish symptoms and help you maintain resolve. Use the Qi Meditation on page 164.

Not all meditation needs to be part of a formal program. In fact, you want to make everything you do meditative so that you can release your suppressed emotions and feelings. For example, during meals, slow down and enjoy the feelings of being nurtured by food; notice the texture, the taste, the aroma of each bite; enjoy the feeling of chewing and swallowing, the warmth of the food energy going into your body.

STEP SIX: SOAKS AND SAUNAS

Detoxifying soaks (chapter 11, page 195) can help you handle withdrawal.

Try a cool sauna, no more than 102° F for fifteen minutes. Scrub skin with a soft-bristled brush afterward and shower in lukewarm water to remove toxins that have been sweated out through the skin.

STEP SEVEN: ACUPUNCTURE

For more than two decades, acupuncture has been used effectively in the United States to help cocaine and heroin addicts break their addiction. It works, along with massage, to dispel agitation and ease the blocks that result from toxins that are released during withdrawal. It also overcomes the imbalances that result from poor nutrition and suppressed emotions. The Shen becomes calmed, the Liver harmonized, and the flow of Qi and Xue is rebalanced.

The use of acupuncture for addiction therapy in the United States was pioneered at the Lincoln Detox Center in the Bronx, and that's where I first trained in acupuncture. The calming effects are astounding to witness: Imagine walking into a room with 150 heroin or cocaine addicts going through detox in which everyone is sitting quietly and calmly. Even those who came in agitated and talking compulsively joined the others in quiet repose as soon as they had the five needles inserted in their ear points. When I saw that more than twenty years ago, I had no doubt about the power of acupuncture.

In the first stages of withdrawal from hard drugs, treatments should be at least once a day, and sometimes twice a day, if needed.

Nicotine withdrawal requires daily treatment for three to five days, then follow-up once or twice a week during the first month. This is done in conjunction with self-massage of ear points or the use of small metal balls taped to the ear points that you can massage whenever the urge to smoke becomes overwhelming. (These are left on for three days.)

Your practitioner will design a routine that is tailored for your individual needs.

MOXIBUSTION

You should do moxa during detoxification only on the advice of your practitioner. For those who have chronic dampness as a result of their addiction, moxa on Stomach 36 and Ren 12 is beneficial. See pages 31 and 186 for a diagram showing these points. If you have any heat symptoms, such as high fevers, a bright red face, or burning diarrhea, avoid moxa.

STEP EIGHT: MASSAGE

Both self-massage and massage by a professional are extremely soothing during detoxification, and they extend the benefits that acupuncture provides. Not only does massage stimulate Qi, provide a kind of in-touch moment, and help remove toxins from the body, it provides a boost in positive body awareness and body-related feelings.

Ear Self-Massage

The general detoxification points are the Shenmen, sympathetic, and Lung Points, plus Stomach on the left ear and Liver on the right ear. (See the diagram on page 179.) In addition, for alcohol detox, add ear Spleen and ear Liver points. Also add right ear lower Lung, left ear upper Lung (women should massage the left ear first in the morning and the right first in the evening; men should massage the right ear first in the morning and the left ear first in the evening).

For crack detox, add Du 20.

For smoking, stick with Shenmen and Lung points (see information above under alcohol detox).

PROFESSIONAL MASSAGE

Massage as frequently as is comfortable. It can provide relief from anxiety, overcome insomnia, and help remove toxins from the body. You should choose the style that feels best to you: the long stroke Swedish massage, the deep energy work of Shiatsu, or the Qi harmonizing impact of Qi Gong.

STEP NINE: HERBAL THERAPY

All practitioners have their own favorite herbal formulas, but the following are examples of those I've found most effective.

EXAMPLES OF CHINESE HERBS USED IN ADDICTION WITHDRAWAL AND RECOVERY

Formula	Herbs in Formula	Chinese Functions	Western Diagnoses
Ecliptex™	Eclipta concentrate (Han Lian Cao) Bupleurum (Chai Hu) Milk thistle (Sylibum) Schizandra (Wu Wei Zi) Curcuma (Yu Jin) Tienchi (San Qi) Salvia (Dan Shen) Tang-kuei (Dang Gui) Lycium fruit (Gou Qi Zi) Plantago seed (Che Qian Zi) Ligustrum (Nu Zhen Zi) Licorice (Gan Cao)	Vitalizes Qi Vitalizes Xue Tonifies Liver Yin Tonifies Kidney Yin Tonifies Xue	Chemical-related damage to liver Alcohol-related damage to liver Hepatitis **Not to be used by pregnant women**
Ardisia 16™	Ardisia Bupleurum Dragon bone Oyster shell Salvia Pinellia Rehmannia Scutellaria Fu-shen	Disperses Qi Disperses Xue Resolves phlegm obstruction	Irritability Body aches Hallucinations Anxiety Constipation Insomnia

Formula	Herbs in Formula	Chinese Functions	Western Diagnoses
	Acorus Peony Ginseng Cinnamon bark Ginger rhubarb		

Cerebral Tonic	Angelica sinensis (Dang Gui)
	Zizyphus (Suan Zao Ren)
	Cistanche (Rou Cong Rong)
	S. biota (Bai Zi Ren)
	Gastrodia (Tian Ma)
	Polygala (Yuan Zhi)
	Walnut kernels
	   (Hu Tao Ren)
	Arisamatis (Tian Nan Xing)
	Acorus (Chang Pu)
	Lycium fruit (Gou Qi Zi)
	Succinum (Hu Po)
	Dens draconis (Long Chi)
	Schizandra (Wu Wei Zi)
		Tonify Xue
		Tonify Heart
		Tonify Kidney
		Nourish the brain
		Calm Shen
			Insomnia
			Palpitations
			Panic attacks
			Anxiety
			Headaches
			
			Use during withdrawal or
			   recovery

Bupleurum
  and Dragon
  Bone
	Bupleurum
	Poria
	Pinellia
	Rhubarb
	Cinnamon
	Scutellaria
	Red dates
	Ginseng
	Ginger
	Oyster shell
	Dragon bone
		Purges Heat
		Dispels Dampness
		Purges Intestines
		Calms Shen
			Irritability
			Body aches
			Hallucinations
			Anxiety
			Constipation
			Insomnia
			
			Also: Epilepsy and
			   hypertension

Schizandra
  Dreams™
	Kava kava (Piper
	  methysticum)
	Schizandra (Wu Wei Zi)
	Calcium carbonate from
	  oyster shell (Mu Li),
	  dragon bone (Long Gu),
	  and amber (Hu Po)
		Nourishes Heart
		Calms Shen
			Insomnia
			Agitation
			Anxiety attacks

Calm Spirit™	Taurine
	Magnesium aspartate
	Enzymes including:
	  peroxidase, catalase,
	  amylase, protease, and
	  lipase
		Calms Shen
		Nourishes Xue
		Nourishes Heart Yin
		Moistens Intestines
			Depression
			Anxiety
			Insomnia
			Constipation

Formula	Herbs in Formula	Chinese Functions	Western Diagnoses
	Herbs: Biota (Bai Zi Ren) Tang-kwei (Dang Gui) Fu shen (Fu Shen) Polygala (Yuan Zhi) Zizyphus (Suan Zao Ren) Peony (Bai Shao) Ophiogon (Mai Men Dong) Codonopsis (Dang Shen) Succinum (Hu Po)		

Clear Air™	Ephedra concentrate
	  (Ma Huang)
	Tussilago concentrate
	  (Kuan Dong Hua)
	Perilla fruit (Su Zi)
	Apricot seed (Ku Xing Ren)
	Morus bark (Sang Bai Pi)
	Trichosanthes root
	  (Tian Hua Fen)
		Descends Qi
		Dispels phlegm
		Clears Lung
			Nicotine addiction
			Pneumonia
			Bronchitis
			Asthma
			
			**Not to be used by
			pregnant women**

Wise Judge™	Glehnia Ophiopogon Polygonatum Lily bulb American ginseng Pseudostellaria Asparagus root Platycodon Fritillaria Tremella Tang-kwei Cooked rehmannia Licorice Poria Schizandra	Tonifies Lung Yin and Qi Moistens Lung	Smoking withdrawal Lung problems Dry cough

Ease Plus™	Oyster shell calcium (Mu Li
	  and Long Gu)
	Bupleurum (Chai Hu)
	Ginseng (Gan Jiang)
	Pinellia (Ban Xia)
	Scutellaria (Huang Qin)
	Cinnamon (Gui Zhi)
	Rhubarb (Da Huang)
	Saussurea (Mu Xiang)
		Invigorates Liver Qi
		Sedates Liver Yang
		Tonifies Spleen Qi
		Calms Shen
			Irritability
			Body aches
			Hallucinations
			Anxiety
			Constipation
			Insomnia
			Also gastric ulcers and
			  migraines

Formula	Herbs in Formula	Chinese Functions	Western Diagnoses
Enhance™	Ganoderma (Ling Zhi) Isatis Extract (Ban Lang Gen/ Da Qing Ye) Millettia extract (Ji Xue Teng) Astragalus (Huang Qi) Tremella (Bai Mu Er) Andrographis (Chuan Xin Luan) American Ginseng (Xi Yang Shen) Hu chang (Hu Chang) Schizandra (Wu Wei Zi) Ligustrum (Nu Zhen Zi) White atractylodes (Bai Zhu) Cooked rehmannia (Shu Di Huang) Lonicera (Jin Yin Hua) Salvia (Dan Shen) Aquilaria (Chen Xiang) Curcuma (Yu Jin) Epimedium (Yin Yang Huo) Viola (Zi Hua Di Ding) Oldenlandia (Bai Hua She She Cao) Citrus (Chen Pi) Cistanche (Rou Cong Rong) White peony (Bai Shao) Lycium fruit (Gou Qi Zi) Ho Shou Wu (He Shou Wu) Laminaria (Kun Bu) Eucommia (Du Zhong) Tang-Kuei (Dang Gui) Cardamom (Sha Ren) Licorice (Gan Cao)	Tonifies Qi, Xue, Yin, Yang, and Jing Clear Heat/Clean Toxin Clears phlegm Strengthens Wei Qi, Spleen, Stomach and Kidney Decreased cellular immunity and humoral immunity	Frequent colds and flu HIV/AIDS Chronic fatigue immune dysfunction syndrome (CFIDS) Chronic viral illnesses associated with immune dysfunction

STEP NINE: BRINGING IN OTHER MODALITIES

There are several other forms of therapy that can be effective in coping with withdrawal symptoms. Homeopathy offers remedies for acute stage reactions and for long-term constitutional adjustments. Chiropractic may ease tension and body aches; Bach or California flower essences promote relaxation.

FOOD ADDICTION: THE UNIQUE PROBLEMS OF OBESITY, BULIMIA AND ANOREXIA

Food addiction is different from other addictions since you can't break the addiction by giving up food. You must use—and use wisely—the very substance to which you are addicted. Furthermore, except in rare cases, the addiction is psychological, even though the consequences are physiological and many physiological repercussions must be dealt with in order to treat the addiction.

The complex social and psychological factors that combine to create a food addiction require their own blend of Chinese and Western therapy, twelve-step support groups and individual psychotherapy. Anyone who suffers from food addiction needs to seek the help of professionals in Eastern and Western medicine in order to create an individualized treatment plan.

Food cravings are yet another problem. According to Chinese medicine, cravings or overeating a particular type of food is often the cause or result of imbalances. As you keep your general dietary log, look for foods that you eat with extra frequency. For example, if you see that you have chicken sometimes twice a day—a chicken salad sandwich for lunch and some kind of roast chicken for dinner—or if you have it four or five days a week, that may strike you as a potential source of food sensitivity. You may want to eliminate it from your diet for a couple of weeks. Once you've removed it, you can observe whether you feel better physically and emotionally.

COMPREHENSIVE HEALING PROGRAM FOR ADDICTION AND DEPENDENCY

Combining Self-Care and a Healing Team	
Evaluation	Western baseline evaluation to establish the nature of the addiction and the physical and emotional consequences of the addiction. Tests for cardiovascular and organ damage, sexually transmitted disease, and HIV may be appropriate.
	Chinese evaluation to determine specific nature of disharmony that has developed: Dampness, Liver Qi Stagnation, Kidney disharmony, and Shen disturbances are frequent problems.
	Other evaluations, if desired, from psychotherapists, counselors, homeopathic practitioners, etc.
Self-monitoring	In addition to following the guidelines given for keeping a general log, record frequency and quantity of your particular dependency/addiction or your emotional and physical responses to withdrawal.
Dietary therapy	Almost any addiction changes how people eat and affects the functioning of the digestive system. To rebuild the digestive system and nurture the Qi, follow the instructions in chapter 6. Once you are through the acute and short-term stages of detox, try the first-step dietary therapy program in chapter 7.
Nutritional supplements	Immune system support is important during the acute and short-term stages: vitamin C, selenium and zinc may be advised. No one should take zinc without consulting a practitioner, and smokers should avoid vitamin C supplements.

***Combining
Self-Care
and a
Healing
Team***

Exercise and meditation	Aerobics if possible, plus 30 to 60 minutes a day of Yoga or Qi Gong. Once a day, go through all or part of the Qi Meditation and make each action throughout the day meditative.
Compresses and soaks	General detoxifying soaks are suggested: steamy tub, Clorox bath, Epsom salts bath, baking soda and sea salt bath. Also, calming soaks and cool saunas.
Acupuncture	In the first stages of withdrawal from hard drugs, acupuncture treatments should be at least once a day; sometimes twice a day is needed.
Massage	**Ear self-massage:** Follow instruction in this chapter for self-ear acupressure. **Professional massage:** Choose the style that feels best to you.
Herbs	Work with a trained herbalist to follow recommended therapy.
Adding Other Therapies	You may choose to expand your healing team to include homeopathic doctors, chiropractors, psychotherapists and biofeedback specialists.

Epilogue

The Path Taken, the Path Not Taken

Seeking harmony should be a harmonious process. That may seem obvious, but too often as we search for wholeness, we put a lot of pressure on ourselves to do the right thing and be good. We worry: Am I better than I used to be? Am I whole yet? Such stressful preoccupation with perfection may lead us to become critical of how we used to be, and we may become more than a bit fanatic about the virtues we have acquired. Seeking wholeness may become a fragmenting experience.

If *The Chinese Way to Healing* leaves you with one idea, I hope it's that there are many routes toward harmony. They may appear to head in opposite directions, but they each bring us to the same place. As the Tao teaches, real wholeness comes when we are expansive and generous in our acceptance of life's (and our own) contradictions and conflicts.

My own path, through writing this book and practicing Chinese medicine, has been a process of healing and transformation. Working on the book encouraged a more direct communication and deeper partnership with my clients. It has completed a process begun in 1985 when I developed my first comprehensive program for people with AIDS. Today, the concept of using Chinese medicine as the context for exploring many Eastern and Western healing arts is familiar to many more people. The New Medicine is becoming a reality. I am receiving more and more clients as referrals from Western physicians, and in the world of Chinese medicine there is ever more interest in working with other healing practitioners.

My search for wholeness—in my work, in relationships with others, and internally—is ongoing. Although I learned many years ago about being mindful and meditative while I am giving a treatment, my struggle is continuing to learn how to do this in other parts of my life.

I want to thank each one of you for joining me on my path and for allowing me to join you on yours. Together, we travel the paths to wholeness.

Glossary

The following terms are used frequently in the book.

Acupuncture: Acupuncture is the art and science of manipulating the flow of Qi and Xue through the body's channels, the invisible aqueduct system that transports the Essential Substances to the Organ Systems, tissues, and bones. Manipulation of the Qi and Xue is accomplished by the stimulation of specific acupuncture points along the channels where these Essential Substances flow close to the skin's surface.

Channels: Also called vessels and meridians, channels are the conduits in the vast aqueduct system that transports the Essential Substances to the Organ Systems. They contain the acu-points that are stimulated through acupuncture and acupressure.

Disharmony: In Chinese medicine when the Essential Substances, Organ Systems and/or channels are not balanced and functioning optimally they are said to be in disharmony. Disharmony can be created by the Six Pernicious Influences or the Seven Emotions.

Eight Fundamental Patterns: Interior, exterior, heat, cold, excess, deficiency, Yin and Yang are the Eight Fundamental patterns that describe the way in which the Pernicious Influences and Seven Emotions create disharmony in the mind/body/spirit.

Essential Substances: This term refers to those fluids, essences, and energies that nurture the Organ Systems and keep the mind/body/spirit in balance. They are identified as Qi, the life force; Shen, the spirit; Jing, the essence that nurtures growth and development; Xue, which is often translated as blood, but which contains more qualities than blood and also transports Shen; and Jin-Ye, which is all the fluids that are not included in Xue.

Five Phases or Five Elements: This is a system that is used by Worsley School acupuncturists and many Japanese and Korean practitioners to describe both the physiology of the mind/body/spirit and to guide diagnosis and treatment.

Jin-Ye: All fluids other than Xue, including sweat, urine, mucus, saliva, and other secretions such as bile and gastric acid, are considered Jin-Ye. Jin-Ye is produced by digestion of food. Organ Qi regulates it. Certain forms of what is called refined Jin-Ye help produce Xue.

Jing: Often translated as essence, Jing is the fluid that nurtures growth and development. We are born with prenatal or congenital Jing, inherited from our parents, and, along with Original Qi, it defines our basic constitution.

Moxibustion: The use of burning herbs, placed on or near the body, to stimulate specific acupuncture points and warm the channels. Used to stimulate a smooth flow of Qi and Xue.

Organ Systems: Unlike the Western concept of organs, Chinese medicine thinks in terms of Organ Systems. An Organ System includes the central organ plus its interaction with the Essential Substances and channels. For example, there is a Heart System, which is responsible not only for the circulation of what Western medicine calls blood, but which also acts as the ruler of Xue and is in charge of storing Shen.

Qi: The basic life force that pulses through everything, living and inanimate, Qi warms the body, retains the body's fluids and organs, fuels the transformation of food into other substances such as Xue, protects the body from disease, and empowers movement, including physical movement, the movement of the circulatory system, thinking and growth.

Qi Gong: The ancient Chinese art of exercise and meditation that stimulates and balances the mind/body/spirit.

Qi Gong Massage: An extension of Qi Gong exercise/meditation that also helps balance Qi and harmonize the mind/body/spirit.

The Seven Emotions: Joy; anger; fear and fright; sadness; and meditation and grief, are internal triggers of disharmony in mind/body/spirit. Fear and fright are related but distinct emotions. Fear is a deep and internalized emotion. Fright is immediate, superficial and dynamic. Likewise, meditation and grief are related but distinct. Meditation is the deeper, more internal emotion and grief is the immediately felt, more vivid, dynamic feeling.

Shen: Shen, or spirit, includes consciousness, thoughts, emotions, and senses that make us uniquely human. It's transmitted into a fetus from both parents and must be continuously nourished after birth.

The Six Pernicious Influences: These influences—heat, cold, wind, dampness, dryness, and summer heat—are associated with the development of disharmony and disease in the mind/body/spirit.

The Tao: The Tao is a philosophical concept and orientation. The word is sometimes translated as *the infinite origin* or the *unnameable*. Tao philosophy sees the universe and each individual as part of the same process. That process moves all things toward unity and into opposition. In the Tao there is no beginning and no end, yet whatever has a beginning has an end; everything changes, nothing is static or absolute.

Xue: Although commonly translated as blood, Xue is not confined to the blood vessels, nor does it contain only plasma and red and white blood cells. The Shen, or spirit, which courses through the blood vessels, is carried by Xue. Xue also moves along the channels in the body where Qi flows.

Yin/Yang: The dynamic balance between opposing forces is known as Yin/Yang. It is the ongoing process of creation and destruction, the natural order of the universe, and of each person's inner being.

Resources

How to Find a Qualified Licensed Chinese Medicine Practitioner

You may write to the following organizations for referrals and certificate information.

• National Commission for the Certification of Acupuncturists
1464 16th Street NW, Suite 501
Washington, DC 20036
Phone: 1-202-232-1404
Fax: 1-202-462-6157

The acupuncturists and herbalists certified by the NCCA meet national standards set for beginning competence in acupuncture and Chinese herbology.

For a directory of certified acupuncturists and herbalists throughout the United States, write to the above address. These practitioners are not necessarily licensed in any given state. Each state has its own rules for licensure. Call the individual acupuncturist in order to find out if he or she is licensed in your state or has received additional herbal training.

• American Association of Acupuncture and Oriental Medicine (AAAOM)
433 Front Street
Catasauqua, PA 18032-2506
Phone: 1-610-433-2448
Fax: 1-610-433-1832
e-mail: AAAOM1@aol.com

This is the largest and oldest political organization of Asian medicine practitioners in the U.S. Write to request a listing of members. They also provide the general public with referrals to practitioners throughout the U.S.

• National Acupuncture and Oriental Medicine Alliance (NAOMA)
P.O. Box 77511
Seattle, WA 98177-0531
(206)524-3511

This is a professional membership organization of acupuncturists, Asian medicine providers-and acupuncture related organizations. It provides the general public with referrals to member-practitioners.

• National Acupuncture Detoxification Association (NADA)
3220 N Street NW, #275
Washington, DC 20007
Phone/Fax: (201)509-7575

NADA provides information and education on drug and alcohol detoxification programs nationally and internationally. NADA trains practitioners in acupuncture treatment for drug detoxification.

State Organizations
Many states have professional acupuncture organizations. There are large state organizations in California, Massachusetts, Florida, New Mexico and New York. For others, please call AAAOM or NAOMA.

• Acupuncture Society of New York (ASNY)
28 Wildey St.
Tarrytown, NY 10591
(800)257-6876

• California Association of Acupuncture and Oriental Medicine (CAAOM)
2180 Garnet Ave., #3G-1
San Diego, CA 92109
(800)477-4564

• Florida State Oriental Medicine Association (FSOMA)
2706 20th St.
Vero Beach, FL 32960-3001

• Massachusetts Association of Acupuncture & Oriental Medicine (MAAOM)
P.O. Box 543
N. Grafton, MA 01536

HEALING CENTERS

The following centers provide a full range of Chinese and complementary therapies. You may contact them for an appointment, to arrange for a telephone consultation, or to request literature.

• Quan Yin Healing Arts Center
1748 Market Street
San Francisco, CA 94102
Phone: (415) 861-4964 FAX: (415)861-0579
Carla Wilson, Director
Misha Cohen, Research and Education Director

Quan Yin Healing Arts Center is a nonprofit treatment, education, and research center dedicated to bringing Chinese medicine into the Western world. Quan Yin's Mission Statement says that "Quan Yin's purpose is to create a new healing philosophy built upon traditional Asian Medicine." The stated goals are:

1. To promote efficacious and affordable care to the community through Quan Yin's clinic.
2. To collaborate and integrate with other health professionals in treatment, research, and education.
3. To promote our healing philosophy by educating on a local, national, and international level.
4. To develop, research, and implement clinical protocols.
5. To ensure that Quan Yin's staff and board reflect the community it serves.

Quan Yin Healing Arts Center offers in-house and by-phone consultations with its Licensed Acupuncturists or its Doctor of Oriental Medicine, Misha Cohen, OMD, L.Ac.

Quan Yin's programs include: the Quan Yin Clinic, which provides treatment protocols for HIV/AIDS, chronic hepatitis, premenstrual syndrome, menopausal support, stress reduction, brain injury/post stroke, depression, and smoking cessation. These treatments incorporate acupuncture, herbs and nutritional counseling.

Quan Yin also offers the general public lecture series and classes, such as Qi Gong. For practitioners, there is the Quan Yin Professional HIV Certification Program and Quan Yin Professional Education Series. Research protocols include HIV symptomatology, Chronic Hepatitis and Brain Injury.

- Chicken Soup Chinese Medicine
San Francisco, CA 94103
Phone: (415) 861-1101
Fax: (415) 864-9653
Misha Cohen, Director

Chicken Soup Chinese Medicine, Misha Cohen's private clinic, offers acupuncture, Chinese herbal medicine, Chinese dietary counseling, nutritional supplement counseling and Asian massage. A limited number of phone consultations are available. All treatments by appointment only.

CHINESE MEDICINE WORKSHOPS

The following workshops provide information and/or training in various healing arts.

PATHS TO WHOLENESS WORKSHOPS

Dr. Cohen offers Paths to Wholeness Workshops for the general public and health professionals other than Chinese medicine practitioners. Workshops include:

1. Focus on HIV/AIDS
   This workshop is based on the Comprehensive Approach outlined in *The Chinese Way to Healing: Many Paths to Wholeness*. The one- or two-day workshops offer a hands-on approach to Chinese Medicine treatment and support for people who are HIV+.
2. Focus on Women's Health
   This women's workshop discusses the application of comprehensive treatment and support programs and emphasizes self-care. The one-day or two-day workshops offer a hands-on approach to Chinese Medicine treatment.
3. Qi Power: Strengthening the Immune System
4. Tonifying the Center: Focus on Digestion
5. Chronic Viral Issues
6. The Chinese Medicine Cabinet: Using Chinese Herbs for Optimum Health

Dr. Cohen will also teach seminars on other topics upon request.

Paths to Wholeness Workshops
P.O. Box 135
3128 16th St.
San Francisco, CA 94103
(415) 864-7234

PATHS TO WHOLENESS PROFESSIONAL SEMINARS

Paths to Wholeness Professional Seminars are conducted by Misha Cohen, OMD, for Chinese medicine practitioners. The seminars include:

1. **Gynecology Seminars** on premenstrual syndrome; dysmenorrhea; menopausal syndromes; cervical dysplasia; women's infertility; endometriosis, pregnancy/labor.
2. **Quan Yin Professional HIV Certification**
   This is a post-graduate professional training program for acupuncturists, Chinese medicine practitioners and M.D.'s trained in Traditional Chinese Medicine who want to do more in the fight against AIDS and be more active in early intervention of HIV disease. For classes in San Francisco, contact Quan Yin Healing Arts Center (see Healing Centers section). For trainings outside of San Francisco, contact Paths to Wholeness Professional Seminars.
3. **Advanced HIV Training Seminars** on digestive disorders; respiratory disorders; dermatological disorders; women's disorders.

Other Professional Seminars include candidiasis; chronic hepatitis; other chronic viral disorders.

Other topics can be covered as requested. All seminars are generally scheduled for two or three days over a weekend, although individual arrangements can be made.

Discounts for nonprofit 501(c)3 organizations.

Paths to Wholeness Professional Seminars
P.O. Box 135
3128 16th St.
San Francisco, CA 94103
(415) 864-7234
Dr. Misha Cohen, Instructor

WHERE TO STUDY CHINESE MEDICINE

• National Accreditation Commission for Schools and Colleges
of Acupuncture and Oriental Medicine (NASCAOM)
8403 Colesville Rd., Suite 370
Silver Spring, MD
(301)608-9680
NASCAOM is the main accrediting body for Chinese medicine schools in the United States. Contact them for more information regarding the accrediting process and status of school programs. The following schools are all NASCAOM accredited as of this writing:

Academy of Chinese Culture and Health Sciences
1601 Clay St.
Oakland, CA 94612
(510)763-7787

American College of Traditional Chinese Medicine
455 Arkansas St.
San Francisco, CA 94107
(415)282-7600

Bastyr University
144 NE 54th St.
Seattle, WA 98105
(206)523-9585

Emperor's College of Traditional Oriental Medicine
1807 B. Wilshire Blvd.
Santa Monica, CA 90403
(310)453-8833

International Institute of Chinese Medicine
P.O. Box 4991
Santa Fe, NM 87502
(505)473-5233
(800)377-4561

Midwest Center for the Study of Oriental Medicine
6226 Banker's Rd., Suites 5 & 6
Racine, WI 53403
(414)554-2010

New England School of Acupuncture
30 Common St.
Watertown, MA 02172
(617)926-1788

Northwest Institute of Acupuncture and Oriental Medicine
1307 North 45th St.
Seattle, WA 98103
(206)633-2419

Oregon College of Oriental Medicine
10525 SE Cherry Blossom Dr.
Portland, OR 97216
(503)253-3443

Pacific College of Oriental Medicine
7445 Mission Valley Rd., Suites 103–106
San Diego, CA 92108
(619)574-6909
Branch:
Pacific Institute of Oriental Medicine
915 Broadway, 3rd Floor
New York, NY 10010
(212)982-3456

Royal University of America
1125 West 6th St.
Los Angeles, CA 90017
(213)482-6646

Samra University of Oriental Medicine
600 St. Paul Ave.
Los Angeles, CA 90017
(213)482-8448

Santa Barbara College of Oriental Medicine
1919 State St., Suite 204
Santa Barbara, CA 93101
(805)898-1180

South Baylo University
1126 N. Brookhurst St.
Anaheim, CA 92801
(714)533-1495
Branch:
2727 W. 6th St.
Los Angeles, CA 90015

Southwest Acupuncture College
325 Paseo de Peralta, Suite 500
Santa Fe, NM 87501
(505)988-3538
Branch:
4308 Carlisle NE, Suite 205
Albuquerque, NM 87107
(505)888-8898

Tai Hsuan Foundation: College of Acupuncture & Herbal
Medicine
2600 S. King St., #206
Honolulu, HI 96826
(800)942-4788

Traditional Acupuncture Institute
10227 Wincopin Circle, Suite 100
Columbia, MD 21044-3422
(301)596-6006

Tri-State Institute of Traditional Chinese Acupuncture
80 8th Ave., 4th Floor
New York, NY 10011
(212)242-2255

Yo San University of Traditional Chinese Medicine
1314 Second St.
Santa Monica, CA 90401
(310)917-2202

OTHER STUDIES

California School of Herbal Studies
P.O. Box 39
Forestville, CA 95436
Phone: (707) 887-7457
Amanda McQuade Crawford, Herbalist

WHERE TO GET CHINESE HERBS

**No one should use Chinese herbs without the recommendation and
supervision of a trained Chinese herbalist.**

For the general public
 There are a limited number of herbs (many of those mentioned in the Medicine
Cabinet portion of *The Chinese Way to Healing: Many Paths to Wholeness*) that
may be ordered over the counter without a prescription from a licensed practi-
tioner.
 The following companies or centers provide quality products:

• Health Concerns
8001 Capwell Drive
Oakland, CA 94621
Phone: 800-233-9355
Fax: 510-639-9140
Andrew Gaeddert, President, Herbalist

Health Concerns manufactures a line of general formulas for the public and distributes other products such as Echinacea, Tiger Balm, etc. For a catalogue, call or write to Health Concerns.

For the name of a licensed practitioner who uses this company's herbs, write or fax Health Concerns. Referrals are not given over the phone.

• Quan Yin Healing Arts Center
1748 Market Street
San Francisco, CA 94102
Phone: (415) 861-4964
Fax: (415) 861-0579

Persons with a written prescription from their licensed practitioner may buy herbs from Quan Yin in person or by mail. Those without a prescription must have a consultation before receiving herbs.

• Mayway: China Native Herbs and Produce
1338 Cypress St.
Oakland, CA 94607
(510)208-3113
London office:
43 Waterside Trading
Trumper's Way, Hanwell
London, ENGLAND W7 2QD

Mayway is one of the largest and most reputable suppliers of Chinese herbal medicines in the U.S. Mayway carries many of the Chinese-produced herbs (pills and bulk herbs) mentioned in *The Chinese Way to Healing: Many Paths to Wholeness.*

• NuHerbs
3820 Perriman Ave.
Oakland, CA 94619
Phone: (510) 534-HERB, (800) 233-4307
Fax: (510) 534-4384

For practitioners and health care professionals

• Health Concerns
8001 Capwell Drive
Oakland, CA 94621
Phone: 800-233-9355
Fax: 510-639-9140

   Health Concerns manufactures a line of high-quality Chinese herbal formulas, including Enhance™ and other products designed by the author. Health Concerns distributes books, acupuncture supplies, and other formulas for internal and external use mentioned in *The Chinese Way to Healing: Many Paths to Wholeness* from several herb manufacturers. Health Concerns maintains an herbal helpline for licensed practitioners.

• Mayway: China Native Herbs and Produce
1338 Cypress St.
Oakland, CA 94607
(510)208-3113
London office:
43 Waterside Trading
Trumper's Way, Hanwell
London, ENGLAND W7 2QD

   Mayway is one of the largest and most reputable suppliers of Chinese herbal medicines in the U.S. Mayway carries many of the Chinese-produced pills and bulk herbs mentioned in this book.

• NuHerbs
3820 Perriman Ave.
Oakland, CA 94619
(510) 534-HERB
(800) 233-4307
Fax: (510) 534-4384

• Springwind Herbs
2315 Fourth St.
Berkeley, CA 94710
(510)849-1820
(800)588-4883 Orders
Andrew Ellis, herbalist, owner

   Springwind specializes in external topical formulas designed by Andrew Ellis, an accomplished herbalist and teacher. Springwind also supplies herbal concentrates and bulk herbs to practitioners. The quality of herbs is excellent.

For a more complete listing of suppliers of Chinese and Western herbs, contact the American Herbal Products Association, P.O. Box 2410, Austin, TX 78768, phone number (512)320-8555.

WHERE TO GET NUTRITIONAL SUPPLEMENTS

The following four companies are mentioned because they supply supplements to Chicken Soup Chinese Medicine and Quan Yin. They may not sell to the general public but will recommend a practitioner in your area who carries these products. Many of the products are superior in quality and comparable or lower in price than supplements available in health food and vitamin stores.

• Karuna: Responsible Nutrition
42 Digital Drive, Suite 7
Novato, CA 94949
1-800-826-7225
   Karuna carries a wide variety of supplements and herbs for practitioner distribution only. I use this brand in my clinic for all the basic nutritional supplementation.

• Natren, Inc.
3105 Willow Lane
Westlake Village, CA 91361
1-800-922-3323
   A good source for Acidophilus products

• Professional and Technical Services, Inc.
621 S.W. Alder, Suite 900
Portland, OR 97205
1-800-866-9085
   A good source for Progesterone products. Although there are many forms of natural progesterone on the market, we use this company's Pro-gest Cream.

• Wholesale Nutrition
Box 3345
Saratoga, CA 95070
1-800-325-2664
   A goods source for Vitamin C (C-salts).

Buyer's Clubs
The buyer's clubs are usually nonprofit organizations established for people with life-threatening illnesses that specialize in offering nutritional supplements at a reduced mark-up. Look in your phone book, or ask at AIDS and cancer support organizations for a buyer's club in your are. Most provide mail order.

New York:
Direct AIDS Alternative Information Resources (DAAIR)
31 East 30th St., Suite 2A
New York, NY 10016
(212)689-8140

Washington, DC:
Carl Vogel Center
1413 K St., NW, 3rd Fl.
Washington, DC 20005-3405
(202) 638-0750
Ron M. Mealy, Director

San Francisco:
Healing Alternatives Foundation
1748 Market Street, #201
San Francisco, CA 94102

California:
CFIDS Health Buyer's Club
1187 Coast Village Rd., #1-280
Santa Barbara, CA 93108
1-800-366-6056

BOOKS AND PUBLICATIONS

Write or call any of these publishers for a list of available titles.

Blue Poppy Press
1775 Linden Ave.
Boulder, CO 80304
800-487-9296
   Blue Poppy Press and its founder Bob Flaws are well known in the world of Chinese medicine. The press sells books for practitioners and the general public on a wide range of Chinese medicine topics.

China Books and Periodicals
2929 24th Street
San Francisco, CA 94110
415-282-2994

Pearson Professional Limited, Medical Division
In USA:
Churchill Livingstone
650 Avenue of the Americas
New York, NY 10011
(212)727-7790
In England:
Robert Stevenson House
1-3 Baxter's Place
Leith Walk
Edinburgh, England EH1 3AF

Eastland Press
1260 Activity Dr., Suite A
Vista, CA 92083
(619)598-9695
Order Line: 800-453-3278
Fax Order Line: 800-241-3329

Eastwind Books
633 Vallejo Street
San Francisco, CA 94133
415-772-5899
   This independent bookstore stocks the nation's most comprehensive selection of both Chinese and English language books on Traditional Chinese Medicine and nutrition, Taiji, Qi Gong, Chinese divination arts, Feng Shui and Chinese philosophy.

Pacific View Press
P.O. Box 2657
Berkeley, CA 94702
(510)849-4213
Fax: (510)843-5835

Paradigm
P.O. Box 16982
San Diego, CA 92116
   This company exclusively publishes Chinese medicine books.

Redwing Book Co.
44 Linden St.
Brookline, MA 04126
Order Line: 800-873-3946

SELECTED BOOKS AND PUBLICATIONS

American Journal of Acupuncture
1840 Forty-First Ave., #102
P.O. Box 610
Capitola, CA
Phone/Fax: 408-475-1700

Between Heaven and Earth: A Guide to Chinese Medicine
    Harriet Beinfield and Efrem Korngold, Ballantine Books, 1991. This book focuses strongly on the philosophy of the Five Phases.

Chinese Herbal Medicine, Formulas and Strategies
    Compiled and translated by Dan Bensky and Randall Barolet, Eastland Press, 1990.

Chinese Herbal Medicine, Materia Medica
    Compiled and translated by Dan Bensky and Andrew Gamble, with Ted Kaptchuk, Eastland Press, 1986.

Journal of the American College of Traditional Chinese Medicine (JACTCM)
455 Arkansas St.
San Francisco, CA 94107
(415)282-7600
    Although this journal is no longer being published, it featured some excellent articles. Back issues and complete sets are still available from ACTCM.

Journal of Chinese Medicine
22 Cromwell Rd.
Hove
Sussex, England BN3 3EB
For American distribution contact:
Eastland Press
1260 Activity Dr., Suite #A
Vista, CA 92083
1-800-453-3278

Journal of the National Academy of Acupuncture and Oriental Medicine (JNAAOM)
28 Wildey St.
Tarrytown, NY 10591-3104

The Practice of Chinese Medicine: The Treatment of Disease with Acupuncture and Chinese Herbs, Giovanni Maciocia. A textbook on Chinese medicine.

The Web That Has No Weaver
Ted Kaptchuk, OMD, Congdon and Weed, 1983
   The first widely popular book on Chinese medicine theory published in the U.S. It's used as a textbook in Chinese medicine classes worldwide.

QI GONG & TAIJI CHUAN VIDEO TAPES:

Larry Wong
Wong's Taiji & Qi Gong for Health
1775 21st Ave.
San Francisco, CA 94122
(415) 753-0426
   Taiji and Qi Gong video tapes, including Qi Gong for senior citizens. The Taiji is based on the Yang-style long form. Meditation and Relaxation audio tapes provide information about the "7 major energy centers" of the body.
   Interviews with Larry Wong formed the basis of the chapter on Qi Gong in *The Chinese Way to Healing: Many Paths to Wholeness.*

MISCELLANEOUS

Multipure Water Filters
1-800-622-9206
   I recommend that everyone filter water with a high-quality filter. It's especially necessary for persons who are immune-compromised.

Great Smokies Laboratories
18A Regent Park Blvd.
Asheville, NC 28806
800-522-4762
(704) 253-0621
   This lab is one of very few in the U.S. that provides extremely accurate stool tests. Ask your doctor for more information.

Notes

CHAPTER TWO: UNDERSTANDING THE MIND/BODY/SPIRIT

1. *A Complete Translation of the Yellow Emperor's Classic of Internal Medicine and the Difficult Classic,* translated from the Chinese by Dr. Henry C. Lu, Ph.D.
2. *A Complete Translation of the Yellow Emperor's Classic of Internal Medicine and the Difficult Classic,* translated from the Chinese by Dr. Henry C. Lu, Ph.D.
3. Jing, the basic life essence, is often said to come into existence "before" Yin and Yang. But its character is said to be Yin. This dialectical view accepts the fact that Jing can exist before Yin and Yang and have Yin qualities, and that Yin itself possesses Yin and Yang aspects.
4. Originally from the Difficulty 38 of the *Nan Jing. A Complete Translation of the Yellow Emperor's Classic of Internal Medicine and the Difficult Classic;* translation by Henry C. Lu, Ph.D.; p. 1202.
5. Five phases diagnoses are not part of what has come to be called Traditional Chinese Medicine (TCM). TCM is based on the Eight Fundamental Patterns and the Essential Substances, Organ Systems and channels. These elements form the basis for herbal therapy and the type of acupuncture provided by TCM practitioners. Therefore, Five phases practitioners do not generally use herbal therapy unless they are also trained in TCM.

CHAPTER FIVE: WHEN YOU VISIT A CHINESE MEDICINE PRACTITIONER

1. Derived from the work of Miriam Lee.

CHAPTER SIX: YOU ARE WHAT YOU EAT

1. Translation taken from *All the Tea in China*, Kit Chow and Ione Kramer, China Books and Periodicals, Inc., San Francisco, 1990.

CHAPTER SEVEN: REBUILDING THE ESSENTIAL SUBSTANCES AND ORGAN SYSTEMS

1. Derived from *Acupuncture Therapy*, by Mary Austin, ASI Publishers, New York.

CHAPTER EIGHT: DANCING WITH DANG GUI AND FRIENDS

1. Adapted from *Oriental Materia Medica: A Concise Guide*, by Hong-Yen Hsu, Oriental Healing Arts Institute, Long Beach, California, 1986.
2. *Chinese Medical Journal* 94 (1): 1981, pp. 35–40.
3. *Chinese Medical Journal* 94 (1): 1981, pp. 35–40.
4. Yeung, H., *Handbook of Chinese Herbs and Formulas*, 1985, p. 293.
5. Cancer Institute of the Chinese Academy of Medical Sciences, "Astragalus Update," *Professional Health Concerns* 102, 1988, p. 2.
6. Zhou, Minxing, et al., "Therapeutic Effect of Astragalus in Treating Chronic Active Hepatitis and the Changes in Immune Functions," *Journal of Chinese People's Liberation Army* 7 (4): 1982, pp. 242–244.
7. Hsu, H.-Y., *Oriental Materia Medica: A Concise Guide*, Oriental Healing Arts Institute, 1986, p. 523.
8. Hsu, H.-Y., *Oriental Materia Medica: A Concise Guide*, Oriental Healing Arts Institute, 1986, p. 524.
9. *Methods and Findings in Experimental and Clinical Pharmacology*, Nov. 14 (9): 1992, 725–36.
10. Yeung, H., *Handbook of Chinese Herbs and Formulas*, 1985, p. 89.
11. Dharmananda, S.
12. Yeung, H., *Handbook of Chinese Herbs and Formulas*, 1985, p. 126.
13. Chiu, H. F., Lin, C. C., et al., "Pharmacological and Pathological Studies on Hepatic Protective Crude Drugs from Taiwan," *American Journal of Chinese Medicine* 20 (3-4):1992, pp. 257–64.
14. Bensky and Gamble, *Chinese Herbal Medicine Materia Medica: Revised Edition,* Eastland Press, 1993, p. 50.
15. Yeung, H., *Handbook of Chinese Herbs and Formulas*, 1985, p. 125.
16. Hildebert Wagner of Germany considers eclipta one of the most promising liver-protecting compounds. See Bensky and Gamble, *Chinese Herbal Medicine Materia Medica: Revised Edition,* Eastland Press, 1993, p. 365.
17. Willard, Terry, *Reishi Mushroom: Herb of Spiritual Potency and Medical Wonder*, Sylvan Press, 1990, p.12.
18. Takashi, *Chem. Abstr.* 98: 212585t.
19. Hsu, H.-Y., *Oriental Materia Medica: A Concise Guide*, Oriental Healing Arts Institute, 1986, p. 641.
20. *Pharmacology and Applications of Chinese Materia Medica*, 1986: pp. 642–653.
21. *Chem. Abstr.* 93: p. 542y.
22. *Chem. Abstr.* 92: p. 51937t.
23. *Becoming Healthy with Reishi*, III, 1988: pp. 12–20.
24. *Reishi Mushroom: Herb of Spiritual Potency and Medical Wonder*, 1990.
25. Yeung, H., *Handbook of Chinese Herbs and Formulas*, 1985, p. 125.
26. Yeung, H., *Handbook of Chinese Herbs and Formulas*, 1985, p. 125.
27. Yeung, H., *Handbook of Chinese Herbs and Formulas*, 1985, p. 93.
28. *AIDS, Immunity, and Chinese Medicine*, 1989: p. 24.
29. Chung-Kuo, 13(3): 1993, pp. 147–9.

30. *Chemical and Pharmaceutical Bulletin*, 36(6):1988, pp. 2090–7.

31. Shinada, et al., *Proceedings of the Society for Exp. Bio. and Med.*, 181(2):1986, pp. 205–10.

32. Chung-Kuo, 13(5):1991, pp. 380–3.

33. *Frotschritte der Medizin*, 110(21):1992, pp. 395–8.

34. Refer to chapter 2.

35. *Journal of Biological Response Modifiers*, 2: 1983, 227–237.

36. See chapter 7.

37. Hsu, H.-Y., *Oriental Materia Medica: A Concise Guide*, Oriental Healing Arts Institute, 1986, p. 590.

38. Hsu, H.-Y., *Oriental Materia Medica: A Concise Guide*, Oriental Healing Arts Institute, 1986, p. 470.

39. Bensky and Gamble, *Chinese Herbal Medicine Materia Medica: Revised Edition*, Eastland Press, 1993, p. 269.

40. Bensky and Gamble, *Chinese Herbal Medicine Materia Medica,: Revised Edition*, Eastland Press, 1993, p. 378.

41. Chang, R. S., and Yeung, H. W., *Antiviral Research* 9:1988, pp. 163–176.

42. *Bulletin of the World Health Organization*, 67(6):1989, pp. 613–80.

43. Hsu, H.-Y., *Oriental Materia Medica: A Concise Guide*, Oriental Healing Arts Institute, 1986, p. 243.

44. Bensky and Gamble, *Chinese Herbal Medicine Materia Medica: Revised Edition*, Eastland Press, 1993, p. 91.

45. Carter, J. J., "Liver Protection and Repair: Synthesizing Herbal Science and Chinese Energetics," *Professional Health Concerns*, 3: 1, pp. 21–24.

46. Lang, I., Nekam, K., et al., "Immunomodulatory and Hepatoprotective Effects of In Vivo Treatment with Free Radical Scavengers," *Italian Journal of Gastroenterology*, Oct. 22 (5): 1990, pp. 283–7.

47. Carter, J. J., "Liver Protection and Repair: Synthesizing Herbal Science and Chinese Energetics," *Professional Health Concerns*, 3: 1, pp. 21–24.

48. de La Lastra, Alarcon, et al., "Gastric Anti-ulcer Activity of Silymarin, a Lipoxygenase Inhibitor, in Rats," *Journal of Pharmacy and Pharmacology*, Nov, 44 (11): 1992, pp. 929–31.

49. Muzes, et al., "Effect of the Bioflavonoid Silymarin on the In Vitro Activity and Expression of Superoxide Dismutase (500) Enzyme," *Acta Physiologica Hungarica*, 78(1):1991, pp. 3–9.

50. Carter, J. J., "Liver Protection and Repair: Synthesizing Herbal Science and Chinese Energetics," *Professional Health Concerns*, 3: 1, pp. 21–24.

51. Weissbuch, B., Personal Communication, 1988.

CHAPTER NINE: METAL AND FIRE

1. From "A Response to the Dao, Charles Chace Responds to Sean Marshall's Essay, 'Classic Chinese Medicine: The Science of Biological Forces and Their Therapeutic Application.' "

2. "Acupuncture Past and Present," David, Joseph, M.D., and Lillian Yin, Ph.D., *The FDA Consumer*, May 1973.

3. Lytle, C. David, Ph.D., Center for Devices and Radiological Health, The U.S. De-

partment of Health and Human Services, Public Health Service, Food and Drug Administration, *An Overview of Acupuncture*, May 1993.

4. Moss, Charles A., M.D., "Acupuncture Stimulation of the Endogenous Opioids and Effects on the Immune System," *AAMA Review*, 2, 1: Spring 1990.

CHAPTER ELEVEN: THE HEALING TOUCH

1. Massage routine adopted from traditional texts and *Chinese Qigong Massage*, 1992, by Dr. Yang Jwing-Ming, published by Yang's Martial Arts Association, Jamaica Plain, MA.

CHAPTER FIFTEEN: HARMONIOUS CYCLES

1. Sandler, D. P., et al., "Age at Menarche and Subsequent Reproductive Events," *American Journal of Epidemiology*, 119:1984.

2. McKinlay, Sonja, et al., "The Normal Menopause Transition," *Maturitas* 14: 1992, pp. 103–15; Krailo, M.D., "Estimation of the Distribution of Age at Natural Menopause from Prevalent Data," *American Journal of Epidemiology*, 117: 1983, pp. 356–51.

3. Adapted from concept from "The Art of Herbal Breast Massage," by Susun Weed, Supplement to *New Age Journal*, July/August 1995.

4. Fosmire, G. J. "Zinc Toxicity," *American Journal of Clinical Nutrition*, 1990.

5. Wilcox, Gisela, et al., "Estrogen Effects of Plant Foods in Postmenopausal Women," *British Medical Journal*, 1990.

CHAPTER SIXTEEN: SUPPORTING THE CENTER

1. Red meat increases the risk of breast cancer, according to a six-year study of 14,000 women by New York University researchers. They found that women who ate two and a half ounces of red meat or more every day had twice the risk of developing breast cancer as women who ate a fourth of an ounce or less a day. What makes red meat so much worse for you than other high-fat foods such as dairy products? Researchers concluded that red meat may increase the risk of breast cancer because of high levels of iron and protein or because of carcinogens produced by cooking. According to a joint study done by the Harvard School of Public Health and Greek researchers, diet can lower the risk of breast cancer dramatically. Women who reported eating five servings of veggies a day had a 46 percent reduction in risk when compared with those who eat only one or two servings a day; eating fruit six times a day reduced the risk 35 percent when compared to women who ate fruit only once a day; using olive oil more than once a day cut the risk by 25 percent.

2. According to *Clinical Pearls in Nutrition and Preventive Medicine*, 1990, compiled by Kirk Hamilton, ITS Services, Health Associates Medical Group, Sacramento, CA, chromium is safe in doses up to 200 mcg a day.

Index